Praise

"This book, and I've read a lot of them over the three decades I've been working with mental health and addiction, is one of the best I've ever read."

~ Mike McGowan- Host of the National Podcast, *Avoiding the Addiction Affliction*, Author, Speaker, and Consultant

"*Incurable Hope* is a must-read. Words cannot describe how important this book is. This memoir is so honest and personal; it describes raw pain in the most vulnerable way. You can tell that it comes deep from a mother's heart; you can feel her fight for her son in every word. This book is very needed—and it brings hope. Thank you for writing it, Lisa!"

~ Ingrid Christine Abild-Pedersen, Certified Professional Coach, Speaker, and Author of *Unmasked: A Triumphant Memoir of Recovery from Childhood Trauma, Eating Disorder, and PTSD*

"Lisa's honest and raw account of the tumultuous, heart-wrenching journey of having a loved one battle addiction is the perfect portrayal of what the merry-go-round of addiction cycle feels like. Lisa not only courageously shares her story, she also provides valuable insight, helpful resources, and tangible steps to help others who will navigate the path she found herself on. Her book ultimately provides hope and comfort as well as clarity and understanding of addiction. I'm deeply grateful to Lisa for writing this book."

~ Whitney Walker, LMFT, Founder of Women Waken

INCURABLE HOPE

A Memoir and Survival Guide
for Coping with a Loved One's Addiction

LISA M. GENNOSA

Copyright © 2023 Lisa M. Gennosa

All rights reserved. No part of this book may be used or reproduced in any manner without written permission from the author and publisher, except by reviewers, bloggers or other individuals who may quote brief passages, as long as they are clearly credited to the author.

Neither the publisher nor the author is engaged in rendering professional advice or services to the individual reader. The ideas and suggestions contained in this book are not intended as a substitute for professional help. Neither the author nor the publisher shall be liable or responsible for any loss or damage allegedly arising from any information or suggestion in this book.

Capucia LLC
211 Pauline Drive #513
York, PA 17402
www.capuciapublishing.com
Send questions to: support@capuciapublishing.com

Paperback ISBN: 978-1-954920-59-0
eBook ISBN: 978-1-954920-60-6
Library of Congress Control Number: 2023903595

Cover Design: Ranilo Cabo
Layout: Ranilo Cabo
Editor and Proofreader: Heather Taylor
Book Midwife: Karen Everitt
"Rescue" song lyrics used by permission

Printed in the United States of America

Capucia LLC is proud to be a part of the Tree Neutral® program. Tree Neutral offsets the number of trees consumed in the production and printing of this book by taking proactive steps such as planting trees in direct proportion to the number of trees used to print books. To learn more about Tree Neutral, please visit treeneutral.com.

DISCLAIMER

This book is a memoir and a work of nonfiction based on a true story and real events. It reflects my present recollections of experiences over time. I have done my best to be truthful in every way when writing this story; however, some timelines have been compressed, some information is secondhand, and some dialogue has been recreated from memory. To protect the privacy of individuals, some names, characters, events, and identifiable characteristics have been changed or invented.

While I am compelled to help others by telling my truth, I recognize that the memories and truths of my family members and those close to me may be different from mine. The intent of this book is to create healing for all, and as such, I intend no harm to any person who may resemble any of the characters described in this book.

In addition, this book is not intended to be a source of medical advice and should not be used as a substitute of your own licensed medical practitioner. I am little more than an armchair expert with a large amount of empirical knowledge. I share educational and informational resources with the intention to help guide you through your loved one's addiction, but I do not claim to be an addiction expert, nor do I proclaim that this information should be used as a sole source in your quest for resources.

I don't know how many times I've rewritten parts of this book, but I feel compelled to preface the upcoming chapters with what I know to be the truth about my son and to acknowledge that this is my perspective, which is all I have.

When I disclose what he said or did, in many cases, I'm really referring to what his substance-hijacked brain said and did or what was relayed to me after the fact or by related individuals.

When I refer to events that happened, I'm pulling only from my memory and my viewpoint on that event. I also use the interchangeable depiction of *substance use disorder* (SUD) with words like *addicted*, *substance abuse*, and *the addict* with no intended negativity.

There are multiple sides to every story, but I sincerely attempt to provide the most accurate depiction of the many experiences we endured.

This book is dedicated to those who, like the lotus flower, overcome the darkness and the suffering, persevere through unimaginable pain, and rise with hope each new day.

This book is also dedicated to my husband, Alex, my son, Tyler, and to all the families who have lost their loved ones to this cruel enemy.

You are not hidden
There's never been a moment
You were forgotten
You are not hopeless
Though you have been broken
Your innocence stolen
I hear you whisper underneath your breath
I hear your SOS, your SOS

~ Daigle, Ingram, and Mabury
"Rescue"

CONTENTS

Introduction   1

Chapter 1	Sweet Child of Mine	9
Chapter 2	Blinded by Love	15
Chapter 3	Smile Mask	23
Chapter 4	The Criminalization of Mental Illness	33
Chapter 5	System Failure	49
Chapter 6	Remission	59
Chapter 7	Love Does Not Conquer Addiction	69
Chapter 8	They Came Bearing Gifts	75
Chapter 9	A Well-Worn Path	85
Chapter 10	Gut Instincts	95
Chapter 11	Raising the White Flag	101
Chapter 12	Damaged Soul	107
Chapter 13	A Lesson in Trauma	113
Chapter 14	Crisis Intervention	119
Chapter 15	Detached Love	127
Chapter 16	The Cost of Addiction	135
Chapter 17	Recovery	139
Chapter 18	Take Care	149
Chapter 19	Healing Through	163
Chapter 20	Mental Health	181
Chapter 21	Family Lies	187

Chapter 22	Facing Facebook	195
Chapter 23	Greater Understanding	201
Chapter 24	Lessons Learned	207
Chapter 25	A Mother's Love	219
Chapter 26	Peace	227

Epilogue	233
Acknowledgments	235
References	239
Contact the Author	241
About the Author	243

INTRODUCTION

Do not believe that he who seeks to comfort you lives untroubled among the simple and quiet words that sometimes do you good. His life has much difficulty and sadness and remains far behind yours. Were it otherwise he would never have been able to find those words.
~ Rainer Maria Rilke
Letters to a Young Poet

You know that scene in <u>A Star is Born</u> (2018), where Jackson Maine, played by Bradley Cooper, finds himself stumbling onstage, incoherent and inebriated, and urinates down the front of his pants in front of millions of viewers during the Grammy awards? It was such a poetic scene for me because it was the first time I felt someone was able to capture the humanity of addiction and the crippling human emotions—such as shame, embarrassment, pity, and sadness—all at once.

I've been living out that scene with my son for so long that as a result, I've spent a decade hiding myself away, telling lies and keeping secrets.

If you're a family member with a loved one who struggles with addiction, I have experienced your pain. I have cried a million tears with you, and I have tried to hide my life, just like you. I've always had the same hopes and dreams for my loved one, who happens to be my only child, that you have, and I always will.

I never intended to write a book, and quite frankly, I wish I didn't live the story I ended up writing about. Yet, here I am—almost as if I didn't get to choose this. It was chosen for me, and I was the unfortunate vessel that experienced the nightmare and lived to tell about it, so maybe others could survive it as well. Just about every one of us has a shocking story to tell about their loved one with addiction. The only difference for me was I broke down the wall of silence to escape the prison I was keeping myself in. It has been a terrifying process, but the more of us who do this, the better it all gets, I have to believe.

You would be hard pressed to find an extended family anywhere in the world that isn't affected by a loved one with a substance use disorder, mental health issue, or trauma. It's a tough ball to dodge. Yet, I still had no idea it would hit our home. Maybe that came from a place of naivety; however, as so many others have had to, our family faced all three in an overlapping nightmare.

I am a middle-aged physician assistant married to a family physician. We practice primary care medicine together in a small rural town where most people don't have access to many doctors, so our breadth of practice is wide and varied and includes mental health and addiction disorders. My mom was a liquor and narcotics agent who became an attorney later in life, so I also grew up around law enforcement and its many rules. I am a product of these forces and, for what it's worth, my experiences are filtered through these lenses, yet they never prepared me for the life story my family and I ultimately faced.

The biggest influence behind my effort of trying to understand the life-upending disease of substance use disorder was my son, Tyler. He is an addict and an alcoholic—and by no means the functional kind.

INTRODUCTION

He is the damaged-human-soul kind who looked for numbness and isolation in his chosen form of oblivion, *liquid depression*, otherwise known as alcohol.

It took many years before I could call my son an *alcoholic* or *addict* or even write those words in a sentence. Today, that ability comes with a level of understanding because it is aligned with education and experience.

Tyler no longer defines himself as an addict or an alcoholic. He decided that identifying as such stole the acceptance of his true self. He would accept that he had an unhealthy relationship with drugs and alcohol only to let go of the mindset that had been holding him in purgatory for too long. I respect that about him, just as much as he respects everyone's personal acknowledgment of how they describe their relationship to substances in the face of this disease.

Some individuals with an addiction disorder say there is a line in the sand when defining alcoholics to addicts. There is a tendency by the AA and NA—Alcoholics Anonymous and Narcotics Anonymous—communities to divide the two into separate camps. To us, the ones left to watch the slow suicide in front of our eyes, we are blind to any lines. Does it really matter what the substance is when it's turning your entire world inside out? Besides, the substance itself is not the focus of the issue; the issue is how the individual and their loved ones can survive in spite of the disease.

The thing is, I have been surrounded by knowledge, experience, and financial means, but there is no amount of access to education or money or maturity that can prepare you for having a child or loved one with addiction. These *advantages* can present a false sense of security and keep you immersed in the delusion that everything is somehow *normal*, or that maybe you can buy your way out of it. I am painfully aware of the disparities that exist and the advantages we had when facing our own private horror show. The emotions and many of the actions are similar, regardless of your background. We all have a universal experience of pain, and when addiction curses your home, you can find solace only with other tortured people who have shared your experience. So here it all is, and it's as real as it gets.

In taking on the task of writing this book, I had to ask myself: *Why would anyone want to read about suffering, transformation, and survival?* I believe one answer is because addiction is such a lonely, isolating, and misunderstood disease. I think I can safely say it is nearly as difficult for those with substance use disorder to navigate as it is for those around them. It's a disease of the human brain, but also of the human condition and of our society.

Although I review the disease process of addiction in an attempt to give it the recognition it deserves and to help simplify the understanding of such a complex process, it is not the emphasis of this book. My point in releasing my afflictions in this form is to share my experience, my mistakes, my discoveries, and the many available resources it took me years to find. Most importantly, I want to make available to others the information and resources I had struggled to uncover or understand. I don't want others to feel as lost as I have felt.

I also want to examine some of the innate frailties and dangers within our healthcare and legal systems. I am not attempting to look at these institutions through a malicious lens; rather, I desperately want to understand how, in America, a suicide attempt can morph into a felony and solitary confinement. If it can happen to my son, as you will read, it can happen to anyone.

INTRODUCTION

This bound offering is not just for mothers, but also for every father, sister, spouse, grandparent and friend who needs a nonjudgmental place where someone else simply understands their experience. I want to share the brutal self-examination as well as the fallibilities of family, faith, and friendships. As you will read, I have looked long and hard for answers. I have scratched and clawed my way out of total darkness and want to share with you how, so maybe you can too.

In truth, these collected words are also an attempt at redemption for my son. Even though our family has worked hard to overcome the sadness we faced, we feel there is still justice that ought to be atoned for by those who have failed him. But I also want to share our resilience because our survival shows it can be done.

There isn't an emotion you won't experience over the many years of substance-fueled chaos. Shame, fear, love, hatred, shock, relief, despair, jealousy, confusion, rage, and likely, most of all, guilt. These emotions continuously fueled the stages of my grief. Denial, anger, bargaining, depression, and acceptance are all stages of the universal experience of suffering. Like many of us facing this disease in our loved one, I found myself spending the majority of time in denial.

Even while in other stages, there was always denial. *How's your son doing?* A question I got a minimum of three times a day from very well-intentioned patients.

Oh, he's great, I'd say. *He's working and, you know, living life.*

The reality was I had no idea if he was sober, awake, or alive that day.

Death is certainly not the only thing we grieve. I grieved the loss of the idealized life—mine and his. I grieved the loss of my son's prosperity, his ability to function without his internal storm. I have been grieving the impending possibility of his death for so long, I don't know what it feels like not to grieve. I have accepted the reality that he has every predisposing feature of an early demise.

However, if I wasn't now in the stage of acceptance, I surely couldn't be writing these words.

Through it all, I've had an enormous amount of support, primarily from my husband, Alex. I recognize the profound fortune I have had as a result of his presence. He kept me feeling secure in an increasingly unsafe world. He wrapped his arms around me and kept me protected when the rest of the world seemed so cold and apathetic, even if it really wasn't, and he provided a level of understanding and perspective that I wasn't always ready to accept. He is truly a rock and a genuine gift in my life.

Several of my patients proved to be an unexpected support system that I am eternally grateful for as well. We have bonded in ways only we can understand. And I will forever appreciate our friends—the ones who never left, no matter how chaotic and twilight zone-ish the experiences in our life were. How can I ever thank them enough?

But I would be remiss if I didn't mention that, at times, my support came from the very source causing the pain. My son and I have always connected intellectually, emotionally, and spiritually. We could hold philosophical conversations for hours in ways that forced me to think through how I understood him and the disease of addiction itself.

My son is a beautiful soul. He will never be defined by the accumulation of his substance-influenced actions. In my eyes, he will always be admired for what he has had to overcome.

There are some who may say: *Why didn't you do more?* while many may ask: *Why did you do so much?* If you or your loved one lives with

INTRODUCTION

addiction, you'll discover there are no absolutes. Most of the time, you're traveling through death-defying and heartbreaking experiences as if you are watching them from outside your body or on some movie set. It feels like a completely irrational reality and like you're losing your mind most of the time. Chaos becomes the only persistent reality, so you do more or less based on that all-powerful heart guiding you to do whatever you can in any given unscripted moment.

That chaos can turn you, the nonaddict, into an unrecognizable version of yourself. It can even make you feel as if you are disintegrating little by little into nonexistence. Every cell in your body becomes directed toward saving your loved one's life, all the while devouring your own composition. You become ravaged by someone else's disease until one random moment when you realize you are killing yourself—and your loved one in the process—in an attempt to save both your lives. You are currently holding in your hands what that chaos really looks and feels like, but you are also getting a road map for coming out of this with grace, dignity, and peace in the end.

This family fought back to regain our life, our hope, and our resiliency, and I'm here to say it can be done.

CHAPTER 1

SWEET CHILD OF MINE

✤ We delight in the beauty of the butterfly, but rarely admit the changes it has gone through to achieve that beauty.
~ often attributed to Maya Angelou

I would like to introduce my son, Tyler. He has always been a soulful human who kept me on my toes with his philosophic and psychologic underpinnings. He has carried compassion and concern for others above all else. This has always been the case—when other forces were not consuming him.

Tyler was born in North Carolina, USA, into a stable, educated, and financially comfortable family. He had every imaginable advantage and was always surrounded by love and support. He was raised to respect others and take care of those who couldn't do for themselves. He was loved and hugged and kissed a billion times to let him know how valued he truly was. Tyler never had to question whether he would be cared for, if he would have enough to eat, or if he would have a roof over his head. He knew he was safe and cherished.

From the moment Tyler was born, he was a smiley, happy baby who slept through the night after only two months. He was delighted by animals of any kind and loud motors that made him cover his ears. He constantly made me laugh—a gift he has to this day. I loved every minute of those years—watching him grow with no boundaries or limitations. He hadn't a care in the world, and boy, was he adorable, with a smile that would melt a statue and soft curly hair bouncing with each step he took.

When Tyler was just three months old, I went back to school to get my degree in biology. It is a decision that has forever haunted me because I've asked myself: *Did something happen to him when I couldn't be there to soothe him? Did the young, tired mother I hired to babysit neglect his cries? Did she ever hurt him, intentionally or otherwise?* Maybe it is irrational thinking because there were never any overt signs of his distress, but as a result of how things developed in his life, I have had to examine the possibility.

His early experience did include my divorce from his father, and that separation clearly affected him. I later learned he seemed to absorb significant emotional traumas from it as well as other events that, at the time, appeared innocent. I failed to see their effects when I needed to.

Years after my divorce, when Tyler was just turning five, I met my new husband, Alex, a.k.a. Tyler's new stepdad, who became a part of Tyler's life he didn't exactly ask for. Tyler has a wonderful relationship with Alex today, but he would later reveal that, as a child, he felt guilty for loving his stepdad in his father's absence. It was a child's way of handling his emotional guilt related to the divorce. With the new parent came another move to a new town, at the point of identity formation.

After a new replacement dad, a new home, and a new school, Tyler encountered a bad seed in the educational system. When Tyler was in first grade, he had a teacher we discovered had been throwing erasers at him and calling him names like *stupid*, *idiot*, and *dumb*, among other outrageous behaviors, such as pulling the seat out from under him as he tried to sit down. He wasn't the only one in the classroom she treated this way, and she was fired for her abhorrent behavior, but I didn't comprehend the ramifications of her actions until many years later. She stole the confidence he was attempting to build at that crucial stage of his development. I will always hold her accountable for stealing a part of my son's childhood and for part of what ultimately happened to him. As a result of that teacher's actions and behavior, Tyler's trust began to erode.

There was nothing unique about our household. Some—especially my son—would say we were rather boring. During Tyler's grade school years, I received from my child all the same love notes on Valentine's Day, cutout handprint turkeys on Thanksgiving, and Popsicle-stick Christmas ornaments given to every mother. We orchestrated elaborate birthday parties with all the kids in superhero costumes or surrounded by *Star-Wars*-themed decorations.

As my son grew into his tween years, his daredevil streak came alive. He expressed how desperately he wanted to ride motocross. Even though he did it for a while, I steered him away from any real commitment because of my fear of the dangers—not anything that *did* happen, but what *could* happen. As a result, he found something else to consume his time. My unfounded fear then materialized. I wanted to be without fear while he was trying so hard to be fearless. I will likely always feel guilty about dissuading him from doing the things he found interesting and persuading the things I thought should be worthwhile—and safe.

As millennials, his was the first generation to grow up with the internet, mobile devices, and social media. Fortunately, or so we thought, Tyler discovered a love of computers. He taught himself programing and editing by the age of twelve. He became a gifted technical guru who, to this day, impresses those who encounter his work.

Right when Tyler was supposed to become more dependent on his peer group in his young teen years, we moved yet again. The awkward teenagers, unsure of their own selves, shunned him for being the new kid. He discovered the freedom from awkwardness that alcohol provided and used this tool to be more comfortable in his own skin. From that point on, he pulled off juggling school, dating, sports, parties, and everything else in those formative years while maintaining the lie that he was always just fine, but his secret drinking began to escalate.

Our life appeared predictable for a decent number of Tyler's mid-teen years. My husband and I worked in medicine; Tyler played sports and attended class trips and school dances. We had dinner parties and went on short trips. He participated in clubs and other outside activities, like Boy Scouts and youth group. Joining these groups was my idea, of course, although he did appear to enjoy them. He made several close friends he remains close with to this day and had a few serious girlfriends. We ate dinner together nearly every night, and he would visit his dad, Sean, on the available weekends.

I was completely unaware that Tyler had already started drinking with his father back at the age of twelve. In *Never Enough: The Neuroscience and Experience of Addiction*, author Judith Grisel relates the statistics are simply not good for the probable development of addiction when someone starts using before age fifteen. People are at least four times more likely to develop alcohol use disorder if they begin drinking in their teens. In fact, the lifetime risk for substance abuse and dependence decreases about 5 percent with each additional year of avoidance between ages thirteen and twenty-one. (2019)

Many years later, I learned just how much he was sneaking alcohol in our own home. He revealed it was almost daily. He would refill the bottles with water if he thought we'd notice anything actually missing—especially later as his tolerance grew—and he drank more and more to meet his body's demands. My husband and I, both medical professionals, had no idea that this was happening. You may think we would be more aware as a result of our profession, yet we were just as blindsided as anyone.

In retrospect, of course, there were signs. Mood swings, especially irritability; school and peer difficulties; marijuana use; difficulty sleeping—but if you ask any parent, they'll say these behaviors are typical. My son also encountered difficult situations with classmates and relentless bullying. After changing schools again, one fellow peer decided he wanted to bully Tyler in the cruelest of ways. The boy used a young social media platform at that time to tell Tyler that *he should go kill himself because nobody wanted him around.* Everyone at the school saw it. The young man received no repercussions for his actions. My son left that school. Fortunately, Tyler found his crew at his new high school and developed lifelong friendships with the young mature adults he met there.

How could I have been so oblivious? How did I miss what was happening right under my nose? I blame my skilled denial and wishful thinking. It didn't even occur to me that he would be going down the path he was. I honestly was completely in the dark, but how does one truly know?

I had made the critical mistake of raising the child I *wanted* to have instead of the one I *did* have. I maintained a bizarre eighties visualization of family perfection. Watching shows like *Family Ties*, *The Wonder Years*, and *Growing Pains*, life seemed so easy and predictable. This is the vision we're sold subconsciously over a lifetime. I allowed myself to be hypnotized by TV, in effect, to believe my son should turn out a particular way. How foolish it is to think about that now. If I could grab any parent off the street, I would simply say: *No matter what, let your child be who they are meant to be.*

Being born a Taurus, the mythical bull, Tyler remained fiercely independent and headstrong. Even though his stepdad and I were always right there, he assumed responsibility for figuring out life on his own. With no siblings and no relatives living nearby, he felt even more determined to make it in the world independently. Working through the hormonal and emotional turmoil of his young years became a private challenge for him that was soothed by alcohol. It took him many years to realize that going it alone isn't really an option for anyone.

Irrespective of all the pre-determined pieces, nobody grows up destined to be an addict.

CHAPTER 2

BLINDED BY LOVE

More people would learn from their mistakes if they weren't so busy denying them.
~ Harold J. Smith

In the summer of 2013, Tyler left for the University of North Carolina at Greensboro to begin his collegiate rite of passage. It didn't take long at all for an attempt at college to implode. Months of drinking, missing classes, and trying new illicit substances made his college effort futile.

As a result, Tyler found himself kicked out of school with the suggestion that he get help. On his way home, filled with alcohol and remorse, he was pulled over by a police officer and presented with his first DUI. We were called from a correctional facility and instructed to come pick up our son. They had released him, and he had started walking down the highway in the direction of nowhere.

As we were driving toward his location, Alex and I saw him on the side of the road, nearly unrecognizable and struggling to walk. We got him in the car, and I'll never forget what I saw: He was pale and small, completely covered in shame and sadness. He was shaking and sweating profusely. He couldn't control the tremor in his hands, and he could not sit still. He was experiencing *delirium tremens*, or the DTs, which is a typical condition of chronic alcoholics in withdrawal, involving tremors, disorientation, anxiety, and hallucinations. Oh, and boy, was he angry.

I never understood the anger until many years later, when I realized the anger was never directed at me. It was only an outward reflection of the hatred and rage he felt toward himself.

Seeing our son like this—disoriented, angry, beaten down, and facing his first of many legal consequences—was our initial awakening to the darkness that is addiction. We were new to this game, and the words *natural consequences* and *enabling* were not yet part of our vocabulary, so we stepped right up to help my son with a lawyer. This was not an ideal choice, but we were figuring this out as we went, without any guidance or resources—where do they even come from? We still thought we were dealing with teenage experimentation. Over $2,000 later, my son had experienced no major consequences. There were no lessons learned and no pain felt.

Now, in my brilliant, solutions-oriented mind, I thought a good intervention would be for my son to move to Texas in January of 2014, at his suggestion, to live with my sister and pursue his desired career in film. I was still unaware that he had been drinking for years at this point, so I encouraged his new adventure.

My naivety, or unwillingness to see the truth, again blinded me to the fact that I was throwing my son into the lion's den. My sister had her own sordid history of substance use. Subsequently, she hobbled along as a functional substance abuser, and I always thought she was doing well enough for herself. However, the supply of alcohol in her home was never short and always in plain sight. When he moved in with her, the damage was quickly cemented in.

Less than a year later, my son returned home to North Carolina after failed attempts at maintaining a job, managing housing, and having an *unexplained vehicle accident* and additional citations for failure to report a crash and traveling at an unsafe speed. His vehicle, which we helped him purchase before we were willing to fully grasp the magnitude of his addiction, was towed and needed more than $3,000 in repairs. We learned years later there were many other death-defying instances in Texas that, had we known at the time, may have opened our eyes to what we were really dealing with. Ignorance truly is bliss.

We again helped Tyler pay for the repairs because we thought having a car was essential to having a job. What we desperately needed to understand was that having natural consequences are essential to getting sober. But when you don't know the language of addiction, you fumble around aimlessly until you either figure it out or your loved one ends up homeless, dead, or in jail—as harsh as that may sound.

He maintained and then increased his use of alcohol that year to a point of self-destruction. When he was unable to maintain any semblance of a productive or independent life, we realized it was time for Tyler to enter rehab. We told him he could come home; however, rehab was the stipulation. He reluctantly conceded.

Of course, here's the part of the story where we all think: *Yes! We've done it. This nightmare is over. He's going to get all fixed up and come home from rehab all clean, renewed, and cured.* We were way out of our league. I can assure you if I had known then what I know now, our approach would have been completely different. It was only the beginning of a long and painful decade of unimaginable twists and turns, but surprisingly and thankfully, also unexpected discovery and rewards.

This was rehab number one. It was a wilderness program that shared outcome data on the results of their program. This is a scientific way of analyzing a response to, in this case, therapy intervention on substance use disorder in a controlled setting. It was designated as a three-month inpatient rehab. We participated in our first family meeting a month into his stay. It was an eye-opening experience, to say the least. My heart felt like it was bleeding the entire time we were there. I cried through almost the whole weekend. If I wasn't crying, that huge lump stayed in my throat as I tried to will myself not to cry again in front of all those *strangers*. They didn't remain strangers for long, however, as the true depth of our connections became clear.

I was the most emotional I'd ever been, but I truly learned a lot that weekend and appreciated the honesty and vulnerability of the other parents there. I heard for the first time how others had been experiencing the very same things we were. I learned that all three children in one family were in some stage of addiction or recovery. We were so far from being alone in this unimaginable struggle. My guard came down in this setting for the first time because I quickly realized I didn't have to hide from these people. We were the same and all facing the same enemy. This is also where I learned my son was up against a recoverable, yet incurable condition.

Several weeks later, when the facility called to inform us that Tyler had walked out, I went into panic mode. My brain stopped thinking with any sort of clarity, and I assumed the worst.

Tyler felt he had learned all he could in less than the recommended stay and walked away after fewer than two months. He believed he was ready to take on the world without alcohol—of course, against medical advice. He had left with five dollars in his wallet and nowhere to go, with his innate bullish disposition. He walked over an hour to Asheville, North Carolina, where he found a McDonald's and took refuge under a bridge.

Fortunately, he carried a phone charger in his backpack and when it was given back to him, he was resourceful enough to find a place to charge his phone. Several hours of fear and chaos later, I was able to reach him and finally exhale. Later, he told us he was nearly urinated on by a homeless man and someone else argued with him about the spot he had claimed for himself under the overpass.

My altruistic expectations are so much a part of my understanding of the world around me. It wouldn't have occurred to me that my son could ever—would ever—sleep anywhere other than in a soft, warm bed. Even though I lived under the poverty line in my early twenties, I was never faced with homelessness or food insecurity. I simply couldn't imagine my son being unhoused because I didn't even have the components needed to comprehend what that meant. It didn't add up. As hard as it may be to believe, it hadn't yet occurred to me how bad off he was.

It's almost unimaginable now to look back and think I wasn't aware, but I wasn't. I feel embarrassed about my lack of attention or understanding, but I lived in the mindset that everything was going to work out. Let's just call it what it is: *denial*.

These events weren't happening consecutively or daily, so there was always a false break in the chaos that gave us a reprieve. My son was an expert—some would say an expert *manipulator*—at making me believe he was okay. He kept me living in this state of constant belief in his recovery and wellness simply because he said he was just fine. He knew how to wield me like a pro, and I was as easy as soft warm clay to be molded. I remained ignorant for many years, and that kept me from making better decisions at the time. It also protected my fragile heart, but that had already begun to erode.

That experience would have been terrifying enough to most people to redirect themselves. Instead, my son came home on a bus with a ticket we had purchased for him—another missed opportunity to let things play out instead of intervening. It didn't seem remotely plausible that I could let him figure out a way to get home with no money or transportation. So once again, we had stepped in to save the day. I laugh at myself now when I think about that. The very reason my son doubted himself was because I clearly doubted his ability to figure anything out on his own. No wonder he felt like a failure. I was fueling his self-doubt all along by running to his rescue.

When we finally put our eyes on him, he appeared beaten down and exhausted. He smelled like a dirty bathroom at a public park. He slept for several days but eventually woke up to his new reality: sobriety without a safety net.

My husband and I simply had no idea what we were doing. Even though we had recently participated in that rehab-sponsored family weekend, we never received any step-by-step instructions—never mind that they don't actually exist. The experience was more of a group therapy session that, while mentally essential, didn't provide the critical tools that parents and other loved ones need to survive. What the experts agree on, but we didn't yet understand, was that he needed to be surrounded by other people in his same situation. We didn't know he should independently find a place to live, like a sober living home, or to start with AA or even a therapist. We honestly thought he just needed to get a job so that he could make enough money to get a car and an apartment. We were still so far removed from his actual state of addiction.

So, he did just that. He got a job, and it was there he tried opiates for the first time. Why one substance has more pull than another, I'll never really know, but he didn't want to try it more than once. He always said that having two medical providers for parents kept him from using opiates because he knew just how deadly they were. We didn't know then what Grisel reveals in her book, *Never Enough* (2019): alcohol kills more individuals every year in this country than prescription opioids and heroin overdoses combined.

Looking back on these distressing situations, I have to believe we all have some protective shield in the brain that prevents emotional pain from oozing into our gray matter, overwhelming it and making life very real. Maybe I was just in a state of shock during this time until my system allowed me to awaken abruptly and feel the intensity of the pain. Or maybe—just maybe—what we were all facing was finally starting to sink in, and I could no longer pretend it wasn't happening.

CHAPTER 3

SMILE MASK

All it takes is a beautiful fake smile to hide an injured soul.
~ often attributed to Robin Williams

In 2015, Tyler came to the conclusion that living with us in North Carolina was less than desirable, most likely because there were rules and expectations. He decided to move in with his dad in Florida for a while and work in landscaping. In an effort to continue to numb out from not finding the support my son was so desperately looking for from his father, his addiction persisted. He drank daily—sometimes with his dad, but most of the time, alone. His use escalated and he was having trouble managing it. I foolishly believed his dad would get a handle on things, which definitely wasn't part of his dad's plan.

Tyler continued his disguise of sobriety, convincing me that all was going great for him. During one of his nights of intoxication, his dad and stepmom dared him to let them shave all his hair off. He went through with it. It seemed to affect him emotionally, although he wouldn't readily admit to it. I felt devastated for him. The loss of hair and one's familiar image can be overwhelming and shocking. Just ask any chemotherapy patient. But he downplayed it and laughed it off, as he learned to do with nearly every situation in his life. He became quite skilled at the comical coverup, using humor to hide so much pain.

The laws had just significantly reduced the charges for marijuana possession, which was lucky for Tyler, who found himself with charges for possession and paraphernalia. Again, the lack of consequences wasn't helping him, and even though we were in three years deep with his addiction antics, we hadn't fully grasped that yet.

In early 2016, he decided it was time to make his way as an adult—at least, the adult he desired to be—and attempt living in Austin, Texas, once again. We readily went along with the idea because it came with the illusion of transformation. He had the best of intentions—and don't we all—but soon after his arrival, he landed DUI number two on July 1, 2016, and we stepped up once again and paid $5,000 for lawyer number two.

I see now that should have been an opportunity to allow him to sink or swim. Playing out that scenario today still pulls at my emotions as I travel down the road which inevitably leads to: *What if he ultimately died because I bowed out?* As parents, that question is always where our mind goes, and it prevents us from using logic because logic says that I never had control of the outcome to begin with. It keeps us frozen in time, trying over and over again and expecting a different outcome. Some call that insanity.

For more than six months, he was forced to wear an ankle monitor and have a breathalyzer in his car. He, of course, couldn't afford the state-issued monitor, so I paid for it, thinking the monitor would prevent his drinking, and this would give his body the break it so desperately needed from alcohol. I convinced my grandiose self it was a smart financial investment toward his sobriety.

He moved in with two individuals he found online who were looking for a roommate. Initially, he strived to make it all work. He truly wanted to kick his *habit* and develop his ambitions. He actually started working in film and applied for other jobs. He maintained his sobriety for a few months while wearing the monitor, but his addiction survived, even in restraints.

He discovered a way to drink while wearing the monitor, and he used in such a way that he didn't have to drive and blow into the breathalyzer for a predetermined number of hours. Brilliant! Tyler's ingenuity never ceased to amaze me. Some called it crafty. I called it reckless.

This entire time, I believed he was sober. I was back to living life, still in North Carolina, and thinking everything was going to be alright—like, really alright, without alcoholism—as if that could actually be the case. He, of course, was lying to me and telling me everything was great, so I believed him.

We want nothing more than to believe our children are making their way in this world. Even after all that time, I was still in the mindset that things would somehow work out. *Maybe he'll miraculously grow out of his chronic need for alcohol,* I would think to myself. Maybe it was just a young adult thing. I could never foresee I would later be holding my son up while he peed all over himself behind a gas station along the side of the road in a completely foreign location in another state.

My son was as relentless in his pursuit of happiness as I was, and he decided to attempt coding school in April of 2017. I was ecstatic and I paid for his classes. I paid for the potential future in coding, the imaginary future that would pay $50,000 a year and set him up financially. The future when he finds a wife at the school, of course, and they live happily ever after.

In reality, he didn't finish coding school, and while making his way home one evening before quitting entirely, while under the influence, a police officer got behind him and began to follow him. He didn't have a reason; likely he ran the plates and saw the DUI history, but the officer's lights came on, and my son went into a full-on, terror-fueled panic attack.

He managed to call me, screaming, "What should I do? What should I do? I'm being followed by the police, Mom! I'm freaking out! I can't pull over; you know what they will do to me!"

It was nearly midnight in North Carolina, a work night, and I was already asleep in bed. I answered the phone in that state of shattered alertness that comes between dreaming and being fully awake. I listened to my son in panic mode with sirens in the background. He drove for at least a full mile at a speed never reaching 30 miles per hour. He even stopped at the traffic lights and used his turn signal, but he just wouldn't pull over.

I kept trying to encourage him as calmly as I could in this situation to just pull over. The police called for backup, I later learned, and when he was finally stopped, all I could hear was an officer yelling as loudly as he could, "Put your hands where we can see them!" I heard my son saying *I'm sorry, I'm sorry* in quick succession. Next, I heard them opening the door; then it all went quiet.

As I lay there, I innately caved into a fetal position. My husband held me in a bear hug, and I began to howl. I later learned the five police officers had him face down, with a knee on his neck and guns drawn on him. I heard from him in the police station later that night. When I tried to answer the phone, I was shaking from my overriding anxiety and was unable to put in the correct information. He hung up on me.

Here was our first exposure to jail and the bail bond system. I couldn't have explained that before this day if a gun was pointed at my head. He had a $10,000-bail posted. I learned right then that I could call a bail bondsman and they would front that money for me for 10 percent down and my willingness to sign over the full amount if my son decided not to show up to court when he was instructed to do so. I signed on the dotted line, again ignoring the opportunity for him to glean a lesson from the situation. I was, however, getting more and more disturbed by the repetitive nature I was finally recognizing. I told my son he had to figure out for himself how to handle the legal matters, and he'd have to get a court-appointed attorney this time.

I had no idea how badly broken this system was. My son got an attorney who had about as much interest in helping him as he did in going to the dentist for a root canal, but after learning what that attorney was up against, I could understand. I read a *New York Times* article by Richard A. Oppel Jr. and Jugal K. Patel that followed one court-appointed attorney who had 194 felony cases at one time—and that was not considered abnormal. They reported, "High-level felonies carry sentences of ten years or more and should each get 70 hours of legal attention according to a workload study. . . . Mid-level felonies require 41 hours each" (2019). It is an overwhelmed system, and these cases typically get only several minutes per case not hours, days, or years. This attorney "would have needed almost 10,000 hours, or five work-years, to handle the 194 active felony cases he had as of that April day, not to mention the dozens more he would be assigned that year" (2019).

Tyler came out of this ordeal with a felony for failing to stop. It's not that he didn't deserve that, but a felony charge changes the course of your life from that moment on.

2017 was shaping up to be Tyler's worst year up to this point. Within just a few months of his most recent charges, he started using more and more heavily. He managed to find a job at a home improvement store before his legal record had caught up with him, but he had been going to work drunk every day. He was drinking on his breaks and at lunch, and when he'd get home, he would drink until he blacked out.

On the night of July 7, 2017, while Alex and I were visiting his family in New York, Tyler's roommate texted me at 4:00 a.m. "Your son is driving around shitfaced in my car. I have no clue where my car is. He won't answer my call. I've notified the police. He has ten minutes to get in contact with me before pressing charges." I was awake enough to call his number. No answer.

I called his friend's number. No answer. I sat up in an unfamiliar bed going through multiple terrifying scenarios in my mind, but after just a few minutes, I lay back down. I closed my eyes and fell back to sleep. I can't explain why I didn't have a complete meltdown at that point. I think I went completely numb. Maybe I was in some sort of shock, but I said to myself: *what will be, will be*. I didn't even wake my husband up. I just informed him the next morning of what had happened.

The next day we were surrounded by family. I was wearing my smile mask so as to appear normal, but I was terrified, wanting to know what happened to my son. My husband's family was not yet aware of our other life back in North Carolina. I just kept to myself and ran to the bedroom occasionally to cry and be alone.

Around three o'clock that afternoon, I finally received a text from my son. Due to reasons he's never fully shared with me—other than he got a regrettable tattoo on his hand while blacked out the night before—he said he was putting himself into a rehab facility he found online. It was in Michigan, and they would fly him there. He said he would call me when he arrived, before they'd take his phone away, but he didn't give me any other details.

Years later I learned that the facility itself was an old psychiatric hospital. It was fairly run-down, and he was sure the religious emphasis was Scientology, although he never felt compelled by it. He also swears it was haunted, but that could just as well have been his hallucinations while in withdrawal—a common side effect. He didn't have many negative comments about the place, only that he felt they were pushing him out before he was ready.

They were going to fly him to Los Angeles, California, for IOP—Intensive Outpatient Program—and sober living. This was one of only three states in the nation that accepted insurance for a private sober living facility. He was thrilled to have the continued support around him, but soon found many individuals working a system to their advantage.

He was taken to the airport by the rehab facility counselor with the expectation to go directly to his sober living home in California. My son checked in and found out it was his lucky day. They upgraded him to first class because they had the extra seats. All the free drinks you could want, and he wanted them. Fresh out of rehab, and my son flew to Los Angeles, first-class, downing drink after drink. He arrived at the sober living home under the influence on day one.

Sober living along with intensive outpatient is a much more relaxed environment than inpatient rehab. You have freedoms such as working, going out to eat, and going to the beach. My son did all those things, and he started using anytime he could find a way to do it without getting caught, until he got caught. When that would happen, they would put him in detox for five days. While there, he was the life of the facility. Everybody loved him. He joked, danced, and laughed his way into everyone's heart each time, so they gave him some extra perks, like candy and getting out a bit early. He would return to the sober living house clean and sober and ready to restart his habit all over again.

Eventually, his repeated offenses got him kicked out of sober living and dropped off on the doorstep of Healing Path Recovery in Huntington Beach, California—rehab number three. While there, they started him on medications for his depression and anxiety for the first time in his life. He was started on Lexapro, naltrexone, and Seroquel. These medications, while life-saving and transformative for some, have warnings, even black-box level warnings, regarding *suicidal ideation*, a medical term to describe the formation of ideas surrounding thoughts of suicide. This ideation became a prelude to his story.

Meanwhile, I was in la-la land back in North Carolina, being reminded by parents who traveled this road long before me that since my son made the decision on his own to put himself in rehab, things were going to miraculously change for the better. I firmly believed this, and hope oozed from my pores. I knew he was safe, and that belief, as false as it was, gave me the ability to sleep, eat, and focus on work. I was cautiously rebuilding my optimism muscle and no longer crying regularly. Like other parents' recovery stories I had clung to, things were going to work out, and he would finally find his life's purpose.

That's not how it went.

Soon after he arrived at the rehab facility in Huntington Beach, he was forced to return to Texas to handle some legal matters. He continued taking the new medications, feeling optimistic. However, this is when Pandora's box was opened, and there was no going back. Our harsh reality was finally sinking in deeply.

CHAPTER 4

THE CRIMINALIZATION OF MENTAL ILLNESS

*As I walked out of the door toward the gate that would lead to my freedom,
I knew if I didn't leave my bitterness and hatred behind, I'd still be in prison.*
~ Nelson Mandela

Your child falls into a deep, dark, cold well. He is alone and it's raining. The smell of wet dirt and metal and fish is so overpowering, he can taste it. The freezing water is pouring in and inching higher and higher. Fear and panic cripple him. He cries out for help over and over, and by the grace of God, his voice is eventually heard within mere minutes of his losing the fight to swim and keep his head above the freezing water. You run toward the voice, and in the darkness, somehow you find the void in the Earth. You scream to him that you are there, and you will do everything you can to save him. You call for help, and within what feels like hours, uniformed people are all around you and your son, who is deep inside the Earth.

Miraculously, they pull him from the grip of Death and put him in an ambulance. He is battered, bloody, and terrified, but at least you know he's safe and alive, and you finally allow yourself to exhale. He is taken to the hospital, and you feel scared but relieved. Later, as you fall asleep next to his hospital bed, you feel as if you are in a dream and are awoken by his call. He's once again in a dark, cold void, only this time he finds himself confined by four wet and marred cement walls. There is a hole in the middle of the floor and a mat covered in vomit, blood, and urine thrown in the corner. You cry and scream and try to pull awake from this bizarre nightmare only to realize you're not dreaming.

Metaphorically speaking, my son had existed down that well for more than ten years, with the walls caving in on him and the water rising, then receding. I threw down food, wisdom, warmth, and love, but he remained in that dark dismal cave. However, there was a particular night that changed the entire landscape of our experience. It was the night he ended up in the *other* dark hole.

Tyler had transferred from California to a sober living home back in Austin, Texas, once again. We assumed we were supporting his sobriety, so we made the decision to pay for his housing. Within a few days, he abandoned the home and started living on the street, all the while taking newly prescribed medications intermittently. He began drinking heavily again. He continued to lie to me, saying he was *couch surfing*—a term I had to become acquainted with—and tried to convince me he was trying to find a job and a new sober living house. With the meds and the alcohol swimming in his brain, it wasn't long before he became completely disassociated and disoriented.

At the time, I was completely in the dark, assuming he was not drinking simply because he said he wasn't. Tyler was a pro at making me believe him. During his maybe one good hour of alertness a day, he talked to me by phone and always left me with the impression that he was doing well and figuring things out on his own terms.

His lies gave me a falsified peace. I believed him only because I couldn't bear not to. Emotionally, there was no way I could handle the alternative story; I couldn't handle the truth. Most family members of individuals with substance use disorder are all too aware of the lies and manipulation their loved ones are capable of giving. My head said he was telling the truth; my heart wanted him to be telling the truth, but my gut knew he just wasn't.

Transition in any form usually dismantles an addict. We later learned that Tyler had become fully derailed and moved into his car. I have no idea how he was able to find and retrieve the car he had left behind before his trip to rehab, although he had become well equipped to handle the increasing volume of liquor he was consuming. I continued to avoid telling any family members around him about the severity of his situation; however, at this point, I began to accept that he was lost. I rejected family members' help or input because of my ego and embarrassment. My mom knew just enough or, at least, what I was willing to reveal at that point. However, she was about to get thrown directly into the fire with him.

If there was a night that could sum up what *rock bottom* might look like—that fictitious point of finality that is supposed to magically transform a battered and bruised addict into a renewed sober powerhouse—this was it. My son's presumed rock bottom occurred on December 5, 2017.

I have always wondered how people so easily recall and memorialize dates of tragic events. I used to think those dates should be forgotten, but I now know some become seared into one's brain unwillingly. This one experience changed the course of my understanding of my son's addiction.

The part about hitting rock bottom that wasn't clear, however, is what happens to all the baggage left behind or the mental health and trauma not yet resolved. In my son's reality, it fueled the next go-round, and this rock bottom became just another traumatic experience for everyone involved.

Everything was spiraling out of control and landed on that tragic night. My son found himself isolated, living in his car, hidden from public view, and suicidal. He had lethal levels of alcohol and a cocktail of misappropriated psych meds and other drugs in his system. Tyler reached out for help from me by phone, displaying his suicidal thoughts to the only person he thought would care.

His remarks were ambiguous. First, he sent me a song about suicide. Then, he texted with me after I asked why he would send that to me. He was deep in despair, and I was now in an all-out panic. I could feel the vice clamping down around my chest and heart.

Is he really contemplating suicide?
What does that look or sound like?
Should I know what the signs are?

As I sat in my home in North Carolina, thousands of miles away from him on the other end of only a phone line, it became more difficult to breathe.

Tyler had suddenly hung up on me, something I was terrified he would do, and I quickly called my mom. She knew just enough to know this was serious; although, her former experience as a police officer never really prepared her for this. When Tyler and I were on the phone earlier, he wouldn't reveal his location to me, or likely couldn't, with the alcohol reaching toxic levels in his blood.

On a hunch, we called a rehab admissions counselor we had been working with. He told us where he had found Tyler in the past—behind several extra-large metal trash compactors in a strip mall parking lot. My mom and stepdad, Wade, drove there on nothing but hope and found where Tyler had hidden his car. The chances were so slim of them finding him without the counselor's input, there had to have been divine intervention.

My mom kept her composure, but over the phone, I could hear the terror in her voice. She told me through tears she was too afraid to go up to the car because she didn't know what she would find, and she couldn't bear to see her grandson this way. When she found the vehicle, she said she saw something moving inside, and I could hear her exhale.

She opened the back-passenger car door and saw that he was incoherent and crying. She attempted to get him out of the vehicle, and eventually he made his way to the edge of the seat. When he put his foot down, he missed the step and fell directly on his face and was unconscious for about a minute—or at least my mom thought he was. When she pulled him up, his head was bleeding profusely, so she called EMS.

I was still on the phone with my mom, hearing every word and movement on the other end. I felt completely out of control and unable to do anything. I was paralyzed with fear. I have no idea how I compiled my thoughts enough at this point to get an emergency plane ticket, but with the help of my husband, I did just that.

When EMS arrived on the scene with Tyler and my mom, I asked to speak with the responders. I explained who I was, my level of experience, and what medications I was so concerned about. I also explained that because of the dangers of the medications, I thought my son was having an uncharacteristic change in his mental status. I felt this could be contributing to his suicidal thoughts and behaviors. I asked that they provide that same information to the attending physician or charge nurse in the emergency department. They said they would, but I don't believe they did.

Tyler was acting in an unrecognizable manner—the manner of someone with a highjacked brain. I once took screenshots of my son's face during a FaceTime call when he was highly intoxicated. I thought I could help by showing him side-by-side portraits of him as sober and drunk. What strange thinking one can have when the world is crashing down around them. When I see them now, the images mimic who he is internally. One image is the son I raised with laughter, joy, and smiles; the other one is someone I don't remotely recognize.

When he arrived at the hospital in the disheveled and intoxicated form that *no one* recognized, not even himself, he got treated as yet another disposable annoyance for the evening. His grandmother was with him throughout the entire episode and remained disturbed by and fearful of both him and the medical personnel who were supposed to be helping him.

Unfortunately, the treatment of individuals with SUD can be abhorrent and shocking at times. I've worked in the emergency department, and I've seen firsthand how apathetic medical personnel can become when dealing with addicts in crisis. I would never say, as a whole, this is always the case, but this night in particular was a true shit show.

I can understand insensibility to a limited degree because medical workers—especially paramedics and those in the emergency department—are sometimes bombarded with, as harsh as it is to say, patients who are not in need of true medical services. In other words, they are bombarded with individuals who use the system for secondary gain, such as for the attention that comes along with illness or to get out of work. This is along with a host of other unpredictable influences.

Patients with mental illness and substance use disorders are unpredictable and especially challenging to manage. Safety issues have to become part of the treatment protocol. It takes a special practitioner to appropriately handle these situations, yet a scarcity of money, time, and resources becomes a roadblock to compassionate care. Apathy can creep in after years of managing these situations.

It's no surprise that an addict's behavior can be completely out of control. In many cases, even trained professionals simply don't know how to de-escalate a situation of this nature, so they treat individuals with SUD as criminals. Having a mental illness or substance use disorder does not equate to committing a crime. And being suicidal, as in my son's case, was a mental health crisis, not an unlawful act against anyone or anything.

That night, my son had been taken to a South Austin medical center for suicidal ideation, an accidental fall, intoxication, and possible head injury. When he arrived, he begged the police officers to shoot him. He told them he wanted to die. He wanted to remove himself from the pain he couldn't find a way to bear anymore. They apparently wanted to remove him from the duties of their shift that night.

At this point, Tyler was put in restraints after escalating verbal back-and-forth. With a blood alcohol level greater than 0.40 percent and his brain now additionally swimming in a disorienting mix of

Haldol, an antipsychotic; and Versed, a benzodiazepine and sedative; his ability to function with any control became impossible.

The affidavit reports that, after waking up in a confused and scared state and realizing he had been tied down, Tyler started yelling about being in restraints. The nurse and officer were both in the room with him. It was at this point that he apparently spit. Whether he purposely hurled spit at someone or incidentally spit while screaming is a point of contention. His medication-induced psychosis at that time would likely be quite contributory, but there was no mention of this in the report. They claimed he intentionally spit; he swears he didn't. There was no apparent use of any sort of de-escalation in this situation.

To this day, Tyler still says an act like that is not aligned with his innate self. I'm willing to accept that a kind human who was suddenly put on antipsychotics and toxic levels of drugs while abusing alcohol used in an attempt to die could have created his anti-self. If it was, in fact, intentional, I don't excuse my son for those actions, but I also don't have the full story. I know, based on his grandmother's firsthand experience of the situation, that the officer was irritated about having to deal with an addict. Even though Tyler was under the influence, de-escalation should have been the tactic used by trained professionals with a suicidal patient, not verbal escalation. Some nurses later told my son and me that they expect difficult behavior and don't take it personally. However, this officer did, and he charged Tyler with a felony.

After his psychiatric assessment, it was indisputably determined that Tyler would need to be transported to a psychiatric unit due to his suicidal comments. The social worker and board-certified emergency room and psychiatric physicians collectively stated that he needed immediate psychiatric care. He was to be transported by a mental health deputy directly to a facility. Alex and I spoke with the emergency physician over the phone that night as well and ensured our son's care and safety was being taken seriously.

My mother was still there with him. The social worker came out and told her to go home because it was after 2:00 a.m., and my mom was barely able to hold her head up at that point. Tyler's grandma argued that she should stay there with him.

The social worker told her many things. She said he was resting, and his next stop would be a psychiatric unit. She went on to assure my mother that he would be safe by explaining what safeguards were being put in place. She told my mother not to worry about anything. She stated Tyler had threatened suicide in front of four people and was asking the officers to shoot him. She reassured her there was no question that the officer would take him to a mental health treatment facility, although we had no reason to believe there was anywhere else he could possibly go.

This is when the levy broke, and everything went horribly wrong. Tyler later remembered he was awoken at that point from a sedated state and put into handcuffs.

The next morning, I left my home at 3:30 to make it to the airport on time. I put myself in a plane seat. Sleep was out of the question. The flight was crowded and overwhelming. I was crying and trembling the entire three-and-a-half-hour trip. I was desperately trying to conceal my shock and my smeared makeup, still barely on from the day before, from all the tears, but it was pointless.

After I landed in Austin, my son called to tell me he was at the county jail—not the hospital. The blood left my body and utter confusion and fury set in. I started shivering like I had just walked out into twenty-degree night air without a coat. I could not understand what he was saying, even though he was speaking clearly. He only had a minute to make his one call and inform me of his location.

I immediately got my mother on the phone. She was in just as much shock as I was because she was told he would be safe and driven directly to a mental health facility when she left. She said she never would have left him if she had known. What began as both a physical and psychiatric emergency had morphed into an incarceration and a felony.

My mother later told me the specifics about the mental health deputy who came to transfer Tyler. She said he was quite unhappy, per the social worker, that he had to deal with another *drunk* in the middle of the night. My mother—again, a former police officer—witnessed the deputies who had dealt with my son and exchanged words. The very next thing that happened was the mental health deputy in charge of transfer decided to take matters into his own hands.

He disregarded the directive to take my son to the psychiatric hospital and instead drove him to jail. My son later reported to me that they had put a bag over his head and left his hospital gown gaping in the front, so the entire front of his naked body was exposed. After arriving at the jail, my son sat on a bench for several hours in handcuffs unable to cover himself and begged for clothes. Eventually they removed the handcuffs, and he was able to cup his hands over his groin. My son started his evening with an impractical, nonetheless real, suicide attempt and ended up in jail, scared and exposed.

I later learned that he was left in a main cell with all the other unfortunate weekend night criminals. Within twenty-four or so hours, he would start the real process of withdrawal from alcohol. This is an incredibly dangerous experience, and even though I practice medicine, it's an aspect I had no real experience with before my son. Heart attacks, seizures, and sudden death—all possibilities in alcohol withdrawal—are known side effects of alcohol seeping out of the blood over days. And yet, at this critical point, my son was put into solitary confinement.

Remember that urine- and vomit-soaked mattress thrown on the floor near a gaping hole in the cement? Well, here it was. He yelled out to find out what time it was periodically because the bright, fluorescent lights were never turned off, but nobody would answer him. He asked for water, but he was left thirsty. He was shaking uncontrollably in withdrawal, but it didn't seem to matter. He was still suicidal, but apparently, that wasn't important. Spitting under the influence was more serious, and for that he had to pay.

Finally, after getting a rental car while trying to keep my bearings, I drove directly to the jail. I arrived during the very restricted visiting hours, and they allowed him to come out and see me through the Plexiglas barrier. I will hold that horrifying memory in my brain for the rest of my life.

Tyler walked out in a jail-issued jumpsuit. He was crying and had soaking tears mixed with snot smeared all over his face, like a baby might have. We sat down and looked at each other as if we hadn't seen one another in years and bawled breathlessly. I put my hand up on the glass as if I could touch his face. I couldn't get it together.

I was sobbing so hard I couldn't speak, yet I knew our time was limited. It was like someone ripped my heart out of my chest and squeezed the pain out of it right in front of my eyes. I wanted only to cradle him in my arms and tell him everything would be okay. I never thought I'd be seeing my son in jail, but that's not what was killing me in that moment. I was there only to see my son, who, mere hours before, had told me he wanted to end his life.

Through his red, soaking-wet face, he told me how humiliated he was being brought into the jail completely exposed. I was furious with the police officers when I heard this, and my trust in law enforcement started deteriorating right then. I kept thinking how scarring that must have been, but I felt deeply troubled by hearing this was what he remembered most about the whole night. He didn't say a word about wanting to hurt himself earlier. But most of all, I remember him saying in an agonizing whisper, "I will never be able to stop drinking." Of course, he would be able to—but in that moment every cell in his body had him convinced otherwise.

Later that night, after leaving my son behind in that godforsaken jail, I became completely unraveled. All my executive function went out the window, and I was left in a puddled mess. I know I scared my mother and my husband. I'm sure they thought they might have to get me to the emergency room for a sedative of my own.

I was staying at my mother's house, and she tried her hardest to console me while I paced the floors, screaming and sobbing uncontrollably. Out of utter exhaustion or anguish, I eventually fell asleep in a fetal position on the floor. I woke up the next morning, ready to fight the system as if I knew what I was doing.

I have yet to get past what happened to him that night, and I don't believe I ever will. This is that unimaginable dream from which I can't seem to wake up.

I experienced a level of rage I didn't think resided inside my being. I could have become the Incredible Hulk while Tyler was in solitary confinement and burst right through my own skin. I repeatedly said that they should put me in there with him with a straight jacket on because I felt completely out of my mind. What happened that night was wrong, no matter how you look at it—ethically, morally, professionally—it was simply wrong. And yet his story is just one of so many.

My son remained in the county prison for the next month without any real explanation of why he was kept there. No one is concerned about providing parents of inmates with information, understandably. He was placed in the psychiatric unit within the prison along with schizophrenic, bipolar, and other mentally ill inmates because of his initial suicidal ideation. Placement in this unit did not serve any valuable purpose in his case. We later understood thoughts of suicide can be significantly amplified while under the influence of any illicit substance.

Tyler told me he couldn't call me as often as he wanted to because there was urine and feces smeared on the walls near the phones. He said he simply couldn't handle the stench long enough to have a conversation. Although Tyler wasn't, I was completely naive about what he would face among the warehoused and forgotten in the prison system. Apparently, one inmate left his water running in order to flood his cell, and this made the rats move into my son's cell to escape the rising water. Tyler instinctively knew there was nothing he could say or do about it. He endured the treatment he was given because he felt he deserved it.

We, those surrounding a loved one with substance use disorder, worry about them going to jail and having terrifying experiences. But are their relatively brief experiences really so much worse than the personal prisons they endure every day within their own addiction? One is tangible, and one is mental torment.

This relapse was an awakening. This is when I became a different version of myself because our reality could no longer be avoided. This is when I lost all control and lost all my faith in God. This is when I told Tyler we couldn't handle it anymore. Why was I handed this unbelievable, unbearable burden? Who said God doesn't give you more than you can handle? I wanted to punch them in the face. I wasn't handling any of it. I was losing my mind and shriveling up into a former human being.

Despite my anger, my husband and I stepped in to pay the attorney fees, this time $5,000 for Tyler spitting on the officer's shirt cuff during the hospital nightmare. We thought, based on what we learned from our past mistake, that we'd opt out of using a court-appointed attorney. The point we continued to miss seeing, however, was that this was not our mistake to make.

After a relatively short time in jail, my son was now on to rehab number four in Texas. He had to be picked up from the jail by an admissions counselor. I wasn't able to do it myself per the court. I feared he would run away, but he arrived as planned. I talked to him briefly before he was swept away into another reprogramming attempt. He sounded broken and despondent but relieved to be leaving jail in the rearview mirror.

We visited him early on, after only a few weeks there, and the three of us walked outside to a stark sitting area. The rehab facility itself was beautiful, and at a cost of over $30,000 a month, it should have been, but it was in the middle of nowhere, close to Austin, with dry, sandy land surrounding it. Everything was the color of nothing.

That day was unusually warm for the winter, so we were able to visit outdoors with each other for a while. I barely recognized my own child, stripped of the soft healthy glow of youth. He was gray and sullen, and he wore shame like a cloak.

He looked at me and said, "I don't think I'll make it. I just can't stop drinking."

I looked back at him and said, "You have to know that you can, that it *is* possible."

I had heard so many other alcoholics survive a lifetime without being in the grips of alcohol. I knew my son had just as much of a chance as they did, and I refused to give up on that belief. It was years later that he explained he drank alcohol like people breathed air. It had become so commonplace to him that it was second nature, and his disease made sure to hold on tight. It had become his only coping skill and his most soothing form of self-harm. I gave him my canned speech full of hope and wisdom that day, neither of which I actually had in that very moment, but I left there knowing that at least he was safe, and I didn't get the sense he would try to leave. So, I got a decent night's sleep.

He stayed on, and as the days and weeks went by, he seemed to be getting better. We would get a phone call a few times a week with an update on his improved state of being. We flew in for yet another family weekend, and when I saw him, I saw Tyler, my beautiful, soulful boy.

I felt so elated to see his bright eyes, full of life, with a big smile on his face. I could see that beautiful pinkish hue in his cheeks as he walked over to give me a huge bear hug. It was as if I was seeing his rebirth—his second chance at life.

Other patients came up to me to tell me how special Tyler was and how much he meant to them. They said he helped them when they felt scared or unmotivated. He was starting to feel what life was like without alcohol for the first time in more than ten years. From our perspective, he looked and felt great.

My son was officially in remission; however, no matter what I did, or what anybody said, I always felt there was more to his story.

CHAPTER 5

SYSTEM FAILURE

No matter what anybody tells you, words and ideas can change the world.
~ Tom Shulman
Dead Poets Society

Every organization, system, or program has its inherent challenges, and it is important to know what you may be up against when trying to help your loved one. The medical, legal, and mental health systems put all their flaws on display for our family as a result of our son's disease, even though we work within these very institutions.

I was on the inside, yet I was forced to examine these systems from a different angle. I never, in a million years, thought they would become part of my world in the way they did. I saw firsthand the failings and disappointments of these professions and professionals from the perspective of someone who wanted and expected to see only the best in these people. I would be lying if I didn't acknowledge my perspective was likely skewed, at least to some degree, and to acknowledge incredible individuals who helped us as well.

To put the colossal breakdown that we experienced into perspective, it is important to understand the limitations we were dealing with. I discovered that it takes thirteen to nineteen weeks to become a police officer. On the other hand, a hairdresser is required to put in thirty-seven and a half weeks of training before they can cut hair for the public. This is typically done over the course of one to two years. Why is training for a hairstylist more intensive than for someone learning how to protect and serve people's lives? Moreover, officer training does not require any initial mental health or crisis intervention education. Officers can opt for this training later, but that means they can always opt out as well. The odd part of the story is that the officer who came to transfer my son was a designated mental health deputy. Did he only check the box for the training, or was he completely burnt out on his job by that point?

Those of us facing the issues of a loved one with SUD need the education and experience these professionals are designed to provide. Dealing with inept or apathetic individuals within these systems felt isolating and impossible. I wanted answers about what happened in the hospital and subsequently in the jail. In a time when I needed more help than any other, I unfortunately found myself confronted with individuals with a completely different idea than mine.

I tried to communicate with the chief of police, the correctional facility nurses, the head of the mental health division of the prison, the many counselors and rehab specialists, the directors and owners of sober living facilities, attorneys, officers, paramedics, and doctors, and I was always kind and respectful when I spoke. I was able to clearly recognize my son's responsibility and my own role regarding our interactions with these individuals, but the kindness and respect appeared to be a one-way street in many cases. The compassion was missing, even though they were in the business of helping others.

Maybe they didn't want to hear about it from me—they wanted the effort for information or change to be coming from the one causing the issues. But addiction is a family disease; there has to be a better approach.

Because I was a part of the medical system with exposure to mental health and substance use issues, I could see there was professional neglect due to what appeared to be burnout, compassion fatigue, or pure apathy.

As a result, I became the apathetic one toward police officers and medical personnel. Their actions as a group fostered resentment in me for a while. Fortunately, I've never been one to assign characteristics of a group to individuals. There are poor players in every walk of life, and we happened to meet some of those players at the wrong time. As I mentioned, we also met some incredibly helpful and genuinely caring souls when we needed them most. I am eternally grateful for the individuals who stopped to listen, offered resources, or continued to check our progress. I am impressed by their true commitment to their profession.

It is only fair that these same systems have an equal and balanced examination. These public institutions also happened to be fraught with fatigue and misuse of their intended services by the public. Over time, compassion gets lost. In the emergency departments, they often find themselves overrun with individuals not truly needing emergent care. They routinely see the same opioid or alcohol abusers over and over—sometimes even in the same week or, dare I say, in the same day. But context is key. A man found in his car, alone, with a blood alcohol content greater than 0.4 percent and suicidal is a far cry from a someone brought in because they overdid it at a bachelor party.

People in need of help from law enforcement are not always appreciative when they don't feel well or are in distress, so the officer's job becomes thankless. It is understandable that the officers' sympathy erodes. It can be difficult to maintain a level of care and concern when days pile onto months, and months pile onto years. When we see the human condition self-destructing due to abuse of food, cigarettes, drugs, alcohol, and immobility, we become desensitized and lose motivation to help. Working on the inside, I had to accept the undeniable reality of the effects of burnout in order to forgive those who made mistakes with my son.

It is tough to do the consistent self-examination needed in these professions, but it is critical. Lives depend on it. There isn't a single individual in these professions who wouldn't want their own family member to be treated fairly and respectfully in a similar situation. It is simply called *putting yourself in someone else's shoes*, otherwise known as *empathy*.

When I decided to practice medicine, it came from a place of grace. I accepted it as a privilege and responsibility and didn't take it for granted. I decided no matter how many times I heard a patient present a concern or break down in tears, I had to proceed, knowing for that patient, it would always be the *first time*, even if I had already heard the same complaint from other patients ten times that day.

Most people have never before experienced the ailment for which they are seeking my advice. Many times, they are fearful, embarrassed, or overwhelmed, so I approach them without judgment, no matter what. Every time. It is a rule I've kept for myself, but it is not universally followed in our current healthcare system. When it comes to substance use, it is quite easy for practitioners to become dismissive and to lump all addicts into the same pool of disposable individuals. There is still an enormous amount of judgment and lack of educated understanding, even among medical professionals and law enforcement; although, of course, this is not true across the board.

The mental health system is stretched well beyond its capabilities and has been especially so during the pandemic crisis. While this spotlight contributes to better understanding and acceptance of mental health issues, it creates a system that is unable to handle the volume of patients needing services. If you add in substance abuse, it becomes nearly impossible to meet the nation's current demands.

What happens when any system swells beyond its capacity? The same thing that happens when you reach your limit. Help, compassion, concern, and assistance disappear. When I attempted to help my son get into counseling immediately after one of his hospitalizations, I was told over and over again it would be weeks to months before he could be seen. We had just gotten through a massive crisis. His system was not just fragile, it was perfectly primed for an intervention or injection of help that just wasn't available. As a physician assistant, I have had to take on a much larger role in primary care for mental health and substance use disorder. I'm more than happy to do it, but it illuminates the need for more resources that are just not there yet.

In addition, our law enforcement organizations are poorly equipped to meet the changes seen with mental health and substance abuse, as witnessed in the mistreatment of my son. Many of my colleagues manage a fair number of patients who work in law enforcement with subsequent PTSD, among other things. In some cases, this is directly related to the chronic overburdening of the judicial system, officers' inability due to lack of training or resources, and subsequent burnout to handle the ever-increasing volume of individuals in crisis. These are the very reasons that Crisis Intervention Training (CIT) has become a much higher priority across the nation and abroad.

I was told many times by both the police and medical personnel that I was just another mother who was unaware of the severity of her child's problem, and yet I felt I was screaming to everyone that it was worse than they could possibly know. I was routinely disregarded and ignored when I tried to explain what I understood was happening. It was a maddening experience. Of course, no one, including myself, had known of the underlying trauma, but should that have made a difference in their treatment of us? And with full knowledge that there was no threat to the officers and medical staff involved, weren't these individuals employed in public service to help the public? You want to know dedicated individuals are in positions of authority to help your loved one when a crisis ensues—and those of us with addicted loved ones know crises *will* eventually ensue.

Police reform has become a universally recognized initiative, even in the midst of a broken system. Police reform isn't about removing or disempowering the police; it is about arming them with the skills, tools, and education needed to respond to the everchanging world and the increasing mental-health and substance-use dilemma. The deputy who transferred my son to jail instead of a psychiatric hospital had received only an additional twenty hours of training to have the privilege of doing that job. I will always believe this individual was severely undertrained and, had reform been a priority at the time, my son's outcome would be different today.

As a result of the combined actions at that time, and while my son was sober, I decided the events were a call to action. Starting in 2018, I went to work on creating change.

My solutions-oriented examination of these systems took me in a few directions. I needed to devise a way to fix these universal problems. Even though I had no control over my son's outcome, I attempted to insert an ounce of control within the broader institutions. I went to work, or rather to volunteer, in various well-intentioned initiatives.

I started with being a guest speaker for Trillium Health Resources, which serves as a specialty care manager for individuals with substance use, mental illness, and intellectual and developmental disabilities in North Carolina. They provide CIT for police officers, and that's where I came in. I came to them as a physician assistant and shared my story, turning it into a teaching opportunity for *their* mental health. I felt that if their mental health was in check, their approach to others with these issues might be more compassionate.

An enormous amount of positive feedback came to me from these discussions, and that gave me renewed hope. The need for broader police education of mental health and substance use disorders has finally been recognized in more recent years, but there's clearly a long way to go. As an example, while working in my office, I was faced with having to make the decision to commit a fourteen-year-old scared, suicidal, female patient to a psychiatric facility, and I called EMS.

Without my knowledge, they called the police, and a large, overbearing officer came in with the demeanor of a bull. He initially wanted to put her in handcuffs. Why would you handcuff a fourteen-year-old suicidal patient who is voluntarily asking for help? There may be some reasonable answers to this question, but there have to be better alternatives. This was a missed potential learning opportunity for better reform initiatives, for sure.

I also began providing group counseling at a correctional facility in a unique and experimental program for incarcerated individuals with substance use disorder. The Sheriff's Heroin Addiction Recovery Program, known as SHARP, is a heavily vetted program for qualifying inmates to help end their substance abuse cycle. The COVID-19 pandemic curtailed that effort, but the program nonetheless was quite rewarding for me and hopefully for the inmates I was fortunate enough to work with. I still see some of them on Facebook with successful, fulfilling lives, and it makes me beam with joy for them.

I took on another local volunteer effort with the Coordinated Opiate Recovery Effort of Edgecombe County, or CORE. Before COVID-19 took another viable program to its knees, CORE had widespread community impact. The initiatives included controlled medication lockboxes and unused or outdated medication drop sites, Vivitrol injections to suppress alcohol cravings prior to inmates' discharge, resource guides for families and inmates, and billboards, community fairs, and community educational talks helping individuals understand the magnitude of the drug problem and the resources available.

I did these things *in an effort to enact the change that I wished to see in the world* and, subconsciously, to see those same changes in my son. I wanted global change, but what I got was individual change, and that is where it starts. People would routinely come up to me after my talks with tears in their eyes, recognizing the changes that needed to be made in themselves. In those moments, that was all I could ask for.

Had the officer listened to the qualified emergency room physician, social worker, or psychiatry consult that night, the resulting years may have gone so differently. That's how I often thought about Tyler's journey in the past. But from my perspective now, knowing what I know, I wonder if any of us had known the underlying trauma, would we have handled anything differently?

A year and a half later, when my son eventually relapsed, I put down my sword and gave up the fight, if only for a while.

We must recognize we all are part of a system that needs some work. As long as we continue to refer apathetically to individuals with substance use disorder or mental health issues with damaging labels, such as *losers, junkies,* and *drug addicts,* we perpetuate the misperception of these conditions. Using these titles perpetuates stigma and stalls any change. In some cases, there is still a ridiculous assumption that this is a condition of the uneducated or of those who live below the poverty threshold. This disease affects anyone; it is as nondiscriminatory as cancer.

In the multiple rehabs my son attended, he was there with dentists, anesthesiologists, pro-golfers, politicians, college students, and yes, the homeless and those experiencing mental illness. His exposure was about as broad spectrum as it could get. Our lack of education and understanding prevents faster discoveries, better resources, improved legislation, better healthcare coverage, more funding for research, and more respectful treatment. But how do we find time to research and understand every unfortunate system failure in a sea of system failures? Must we really wait until we are affected personally for motivation to act?

Some studies suggest that one out of every eight adults has a clinically diagnosable addiction potential lying in wait. Maybe it's just easier to vilify people to explain away their affliction, but it's truly our lack of education and understanding that is preventing faster discoveries in this particular field of medicine.

To understand and educate, we, the unfortunate ambassadors, need to use more respectful language. We know our words matter. As a start, change *addiction* to *substance use disorder* and *clean* to *in remission*. It helps to shift the mindset of the person hearing these terms and begin to deteriorate the stigma.

There will always be more work to do, at least in my lifetime. I will continue to work on reform, education, and self-improvement because every day is a chance for change. I can't *fix* my son, or these large ingrained systems per se, but I can participate in doing the small things daily that help promote larger change. I encourage you to do the same. Every day I have intimate conversations with patients about these life challenges. I am grateful for that platform to instill education and information when I can. When pulling back and examining the life experience I've been handed, it has given me a sense of purpose. And a sense of purpose is what you, the family member, can benefit from for your own recovery.

CHAPTER 6

REMISSION

When there is no hope, there can be no endeavor.
~ Samuel Johnson

For two glorious years, Tyler maintained his sobriety. During that time, I gained many rewarding experiences. That time was absolutely wonderful. I could renew my relationship with the son I had formerly known. Alex and I cautiously allowed ourselves to experience life again. We socialized and traveled. We laughed. And we felt there was a chance Tyler would actually make it.

When I visited Tyler in Austin for his birthday, we stopped at a mall to run some errands. Before I could get out of the car, he said he needed to say his amends to me.

"You don't have to do that," I started to say, but he cut me off.

"Let me finish," he said. He authentically apologized directly from the depths of his heart about what he had put me through. He recognized his contribution to my sadness and despair. He didn't want to be responsible for that anymore. After saying everything he needed to say, he went on to ask me to be very candid about what he put me through in my own words. It was one of the more vulnerable moments in my life.

After a long pause, I took a deep breath and said, "Your addiction—not you, but your addiction—nearly destroyed my marriage. Alex and I have a strong marriage, but I am trying to manage an insurmountable amount of guilt for putting him through my anger and depression."

I explained I was pushing Alex away because I thought I was shielding him from pain, but pushing him away hurt him even more. I emphasized I was sad about what Alex had been put through; he had to watch me collapse in pain that he couldn't take away. He felt helpless to help me or himself, and, in his mind, this went against everything a husband is supposed to do for his family. I went on to say we were doing better, but we had so much healing to do ourselves, and it would take time.

I then cautiously told Tyler the most difficult truth of my life: I told him I had contemplated the value of my own life because I couldn't handle the pain of his disease anymore. I told him how I remembered the very evening when I got to a place of utter darkness.

I never came to formulate how I would do anything to hurt myself, but I had spiraled into the depths of my despair, and just couldn't see how to make life better. I had never had a thought like that before that night or since, yet it was there. It had crossed my mind, and that's an unimaginable idea to hold in one's head, even for a second.

"I can't watch you slowly commit your own suicide with alcohol," I said. "I hit my lowest point, but I am so grateful in this moment to be sitting here with you, seeing life with all its potential for you." At this point, we were both crying.

We got out of the car, and in front of the consumer's paradise, with grateful tears running down our cheeks, we gave each other a very long and much needed hug, unaware of the shoppers walking around us trying to get into the stores.

After rehab and Intensive Outpatient Treatment in that dual diagnosis facility in Texas, where my son got real help for what felt like the first time, he moved into another sober living home he had located through one of his friends at rehab. Dual diagnosis facilities address both substance use disorders and mental health. It was not just an addiction rehab center, and that was critical for Tyler.

The sober living home was a tightly run ship. All rules had to be abided with no exceptions, or you would be thrown out on the spot. My son participated with the other guys in AA, hospital in-services, sponsorship, working out, and job hunting. He even took care of some face-to-face amends head on.

His first amends was with his old job at the home improvement store. He went in and told them he had been drunk most days on the job there, and he was eternally sorry for his behavior. Somehow, he had never made any critical errors while on the clock; nonetheless, he knew there was always that lurking potential. They graciously thanked him for his honesty and gave him hugs and congratulations for his sobriety.

Next, he went to a grocery store, where he had stolen several bottles of wine. He admitted to his theft and said he would humbly accept any consequences. He knew they could call the police or that they could make him pay with interest, but instead, they also congratulated him on his sobriety and sincerely thanked him for his honesty. He tried to pay them back, but they wouldn't take it. I marvel to this day at the generosity of these major companies and the individuals who approached his admission of guilt with grace and forgiveness.

Lastly, my son had done something under the influence that he was so ashamed of, and he knew he needed to come clean. Tyler had spray-painted obscenities on the front of a bank in the middle of the night while in a near blacked-out state. It was extremely damaging and likely very expensive to clean up. My son walked into the bank and asked to speak with the manager. He was forthcoming and did not mince words. He told them he was responsible for the damage done to their building a year before. He explained why he did it, and how he was now reformed. He apologized profusely and said he would be willing to pay any damages as they saw fit. His words evidently drew several of the female workers at the bank around the manager. He was terrified they would call the police and he would be taken back to jail.

Instead, the manager took him into the office and talked to him. She asked him about his life and soon after, she started to cry and asked him if she could give him a hug. He exposed the rawest, most difficult side of his human condition to these people, and instead of chastising him, they wrapped their arms around him and told him they admired him and that he was an incredible inspiration.

For a mom, I don't think there are enough words to express my gratitude. I am in awe of their grace and compassion. The acceptance and forgiveness by individuals indirectly affected by my son compared to the individuals in the hospital who treated my son as less than human enabled me to hold on to good in the world. The very people who didn't have to treat my son with respect after what he had done chose compassion, and the people who went into a profession underscored by caring chose inhumanity. I will always remain baffled by this.

After about six months, Tyler was promoted to assistant manager at the sober living home. With that came more responsibility, but it also diminished his rent, so it was a win-win for him. He relished his new responsibilities and did a great job. I felt these things would give him the fortitude to remain in remission. However, as the story of addiction often goes, toward the end of those two blissful years, two major shifts in the tectonic plates took hold.

Not surprisingly, the first one involved a woman he met. Tyler held his position with her on maintaining their sobriety together, but she played him, and he tanked emotionally. She had been cheating on him and using her *drug of choice*, or DOC, with regularity. She was young and had mental health challenges, so it didn't start out with ideal circumstances. They broke up and that broke him. There are rules about dating in early sobriety and it is strongly recommended to wait at least a year before putting yourself to the relationship test. He didn't think that was necessary despite all the warning signs. I felt concerned, but I tried to remain supportive because at the time, I hoped love would be an antidote for addiction.

The second shift occurred when he was promoted to manager. At that point, he had to change his residence and live with all new guys. Change has never been easy for Tyler, but with the additional burden of addiction, change can be catastrophic. It proved to be just that. He called me repeatedly, saying he was unhappy with his situation. I could hear him falling off the proverbial cliff. He sounded more and more desperate and discontented as the days passed in his new house. I think the final straw came when he had to kick a guy out on to the street for using Kratom. Tyler felt so responsible for making someone homeless. In a matter of days, he just simply walked away, leaving a good portion of his belongings behind. He started drinking again.

I had recognized signs that my son was losing his will to stay sober. He would complain about AA or say he wasn't going to go as frequently. Then he would tell me about others' relapses or how much worse off they were than he. "No one can talk about anything but their sobriety," he complained.

Tyler wanted so desperately to know what it felt like to have what he called "a normal conversation," absent of substance talk, that it became his number one goal. All of this ultimately opened the door to his relapse. I see now that it was as if he had given himself permission to numb out once again.

As is the case for many parents in that situation, I felt it coming, but I was still devastated—and that might not even be a strong enough word for how I truly felt. I wish I had seen the writing on the wall so much sooner.

The owner of the sober living home called me to let me know what had happened. I immediately backslid into the frenzied, terrified mother I had previously learned how to be. I scouted out his location and status. I reached out to everyone I knew to put them on the all-out manhunt. I wasn't ready to let things play out as they could have naturally. We used what technology we could to find his location, and I was able to talk to him within several hours of his departure. He needed to flee as addicts do, because his brain couldn't handle the surging stress any longer. I screamed and yelled at God for putting us all back in this living nightmare once again. I cried and cried for days.

He continued to get around Austin on his motorbike, always the nomad at heart, always fleeing from any semblance of feelings. Within a day, he found a way to couch surf once again. Within the first few days, several of his *friends*, a term I use loosely, threw him out, but he was able to find a more permanent couch at an old friend's apartment. This was the same friend who, months before, had been ready to turn him over to the police and had texted me at 4:00 a.m. to inform me of such. I couldn't believe Tyler would do this, but he lied and said he was getting his life together on his own terms. I still had space in my brain that believed him, but it was what I wanted to believe instead of what was true.

By late 2019, my sanity, my job, and my marriage all required that I start pulling away from Tyler in an attempt to salvage what was left of my life. But it was likely just my body shutting down to withstand the pain. I could not see how I would be able to keep going this time. How could I hold on to hope when his attempt to maintain sobriety failed in the way that it did? He relapsed after two years of abstaining from alcohol, or any other drugs for that matter, so I followed suit and relapsed into my pain again.

I didn't understand that he was merely in remission and that relapse is a part of the process. I still hadn't fully accepted this to be an incurable lifelong disease he would have to face—we all would have to face.

Within a relatively short time, while still sleeping on a couch and drinking heavily, he landed a landscaping job. He worked with guys who were typically high on any given day from any given substance. Tyler was drinking toxic quantities in a short time, and his world began to fall down around him, as it always had.

I was still in North Carolina. I struggled with whether to fly to Texas again. I had flown there in response to his crises dozens of times because of his choices. If I stepped in this time, would I be enabling? But if I didn't, would I be abandoning him?

I had to accept that sometimes, holding on does more damage than letting go. Also, my son maintained contact with me almost every day. I believe it was a manipulation tactic to keep me hoping. I lived there, cautiously believing he would make a dramatic shift toward a well-meaning life. Because this fantasy fit my expectations, I stayed starry-eyed and in denial. All I know is that he was not able to avoid the consequences of ignoring reality.

The weeks went by, and the police were called to the apartment multiple times because of all the screaming and yelling. I knew things were on the verge of imploding between him and his roommate. While intoxicated at a near-black-out level, my son brilliantly decided to text with his roommate's girlfriend while making suggestive advances toward her.

After hours of fighting, she kicked Tyler out of the apartment. Once again, he was drunk and homeless. I would not have known any of this had happened if I had not answered my phone when he repeatedly called me that night. I was feeding into my own addiction by being right where he wanted me to be. I was responding to his cry for help each and every time he felt he needed to place his burdens on my shoulders. I was constantly letting him dictate my emotional state. When I just couldn't take it any longer, I put myself in bed in the fetal position and cried my heart out. I prayed in that accusatory tone to God and told Him to fix the problem. I laugh at myself for that now.

REMISSION

That night, Tyler eventually called a familiar friend, Dean, for help. As his friends who loved him dearly always did, Dean told Tyler to stay where he was. Dean would pick him up as soon as possible and help him clean and sober up. Tyler's friend did what he said he would and brought him to his home.

Tyler, in the company of his friend, a gentleman nearly my own age, called me so we could all talk and try to come up with a reasonable solution. It was always such an uncomfortable feeling to have to talk to the people trying to help clean up Tyler's mess. I was embarrassed for not being there to take care of our own family's personal disaster, but at the same time, so angry that I was always expected to be that person for him. I never knew how to have that awkward conversation with people trying to help. Did they know what they were really dealing with? Had they ever been up close and personal to someone as bad off as my son was? Did they really understand the complexity of the situation?

We all reluctantly decided that, due to Tyler's homelessness, joblessness, and lack of a single penny in his pocket, we would fly him back to North Carolina where he could again get into the grips of my infinite wisdom. As low as he was, he was hesitant but out of alcohol, so he reluctantly agreed. Tyler was starting to panic as the walls around him were closing in, and his anxiety was causing crushing chest pain. As a result, that fear rose to the point where he swore he had COVID-19. He did not.

Later that day, airlines announced their flights would become limited because the pandemic had reached global proportions. He was on one of the last standard commercial flights before the world seemed to shut down. This was March of 2020.

CHAPTER 7

LOVE DOES NOT CONQUER ADDICTION

Be careful. Manipulation can feel like love.
~ Unknown

When Tyler arrived in North Carolina, we made it abundantly clear that he would not be able to drink in our home under any circumstances. The tradeoff? We would help him get back on his feet.

I returned to the simplistic thought that if he had a home, a car, a job, and some money, he'd have the makings of sobriety. Accumulating these things doesn't cure addiction, but I had yet to integrate that truth. My husband, my son, and I legitimately tried for several months. Tyler appeared to be coming along, but I continued to fear the lying, deceiving, and manipulating that exists with addicts. I think this is why people associate moral failing with addicts, even though that's just not what addiction is about.

After several months, Tyler became restless. Opportunities weren't falling into his lap, and the pandemic was taking hold, so as Tyler had before, we *all* now felt the walls closing in.

He was also continually trying to avoid his past. We assumed the past he was trying to avoid included his own mistakes and shame related to years of alcohol induced missteps. We recognized a pattern over the previous few years in which he would spontaneously disappear and abandon everyone and everything he knew, although his trauma was determined to keep up with him. It was his shadow, his tormentor—always ready to pounce. We remained in the dark about what was trapped within him under his protective shell.

Tyler was trying to find work, so we offered him some money in exchange for painting our garage doors. He had remained sober since his arrival, and things appeared to be going along really well, so we felt secure in that choice at the time. He managed to buy a vehicle on his own with the government-issued pandemic relief check and was still working on his first semester in art school, which ended up online because of the pandemic. We had another injection of hope, and we were riding high on this recent flurry of opportunities.

We drove home from the beach in good spirits one night after the garage doors were nearly done, anticipating sharing takeout dinner with Tyler. On the way, we tried to call him to let him know our ETA and where to pick up the food. He didn't answer. I texted him and said to give us a call back so we could coordinate. He didn't text us. When we got home, his truck wasn't there. My first thought was simply that he'd gone to pick up the food without letting us know, but when we walked in and looked around for him, we realized he had vanished. He had left us a note apologizing for his abrupt abandonment and stated he couldn't do it anymore; he loved us and thanked us.

I howled when I realized what happened. Alex wrapped his arms around me and tried to console me, but I couldn't stop crying for hours. I just felt so used and dismissed. What Tyler did or didn't do was never about us. It's the mental torment of the addicted person that makes them do the misguided things they do, but that's not how I felt in that moment. Resentment and numbness became my home once again.

Two days later, he called. By then I had settled down and was just angry. He apologized again and said he needed to get out from under us. I later learned that he had been drinking heavily at that time but forgot to mention that when we talked. He drove himself across the country and into Random Town, Colorado, to meet some friends he had become acquainted with through Instagram. He called to tell me that their meeting was very short lived, so he was on his way south, back to Austin, where he knew the best and worst of his life had already been sewn. He never told me otherwise, but my guess is the Colorado friends had taken one good look and smell of Tyler and decided they had other things to do.

After he just left us behind, I didn't understand why he called me—or why I answered the phone every time he did. I mean, of course, I wanted to hear from him and know where he was and that he was still alive, but it hurt. I realized he was codependent with me, and I was with him. He needed to feed off me, and I needed to know I was there for him. It was so unhealthy. From our vantage point, however, no one could tell us we were doing anything wrong, let alone being *codependent*. I started reading Melody Beattie's *Codependent No More* for the second time after he left. Even though the book had been planting valuable seeds, those seeds wouldn't take root until I had surrendered, almost a year later. My empathy for his pain, the same empathy he had for the world, kept me bound to him.

I was so bewildered and, honestly, terrified by his choices. Why was he driving back to Texas in the first place? He was just running from everything and nothing, so he kept driving. He was bleary eyed and sleep deprived, but he had nowhere to go. He was talking to me daily because he needed to know someone was there to hear how miserable he was. He described a desolate landscape, almost as desolate as I was feeling, that was making him feel more isolated than he ever had, but he decided to keep driving south to stay with an old friend he knew from the film business.

I got to know Tyler's friend, James, and his wife, Candace, from years past. I had James's phone number, so he kept me up to date when he could after Tyler arrived there, but it wasn't his job to do so. James became a source of encouragement for both Tyler and me over the next few days. He told me he too had a dim view of the future when he was about Tyler's age.

With Tyler safe at his house, James shared a valuable story to attempt to give me some comfort, I suppose. He said, "When I was young and lost, I moved to a jungle in Hawaii, built myself a grass hut to live in, gathered water from waterfalls, ate a bunch of fruit, and didn't speak to another soul for months." He went on to say, "I was living like there was no tomorrow, or that it didn't matter what I did because I felt like there was no purpose in life. However, the tomorrows did keep coming, and I knew they would continue to pile up, so I came out of the jungle." He said, "I'll try to help Tyler see the jungle for what it is and help him cut his own path through it. Tyler has a good heart, and he's super smart. I'll try my damnedest to lend T the proper sort of inspiration."

James told me he knew of Tyler's troubles because he suffered from a similar affliction in the past. He happened to have an old Airstream in his back yard that he let wayward individuals use when they were down on their luck. He offered it to Tyler.

Once Tyler got set up, he escalated his drinking to match his level of newfound isolation. We talked when he would answer the phone. Maybe I should have just stopped reaching out to him, but I could picture him alone in that Airstream drinking himself into oblivion, and it turned me into that completely dysfunctional human only people with an addicted loved one can relate to. I couldn't sleep or eat or even pet my dogs, which sounds kind of unusual, but my dogs were my biggest source of comfort at times. I was useless because my son was somewhere feeding his depression with cheap, store-bought poison. I became hopelessly depressed, and yet, somehow, we still had more suffering to confront.

CHAPTER 8

THEY CAME BEARING GIFTS

The truth which makes men free is for the most part the truth which men prefer not to hear.
~ Herbert Agar

I always asked myself: *Why don't I fly there to rescue him?* It's a complex situation. He would routinely run when I would try to find him, which had the potential to push him deeper into hiding and isolation, and that terrified me. When I didn't look for him, he would at least talk to me by phone daily, so I always knew where he was for the most part. I knew I could potentially get the police to him as long as I knew his location.

I knew I had to let him come to terms with what he was doing on his own, not assert my power over him, which never works. It's a mind game—a tug-of-war that should not have to be a part of parenting. I never imagined I'd be making these gut-wrenching decisions about my son's life. I couldn't have imagined any of this. Only fellow parents or loved ones of someone with substance use disorder understand this internal fight within us.

With James's help, I eventually convinced Tyler to drive home and start again. The past would be forgotten, and we would simply move forward. He could only get in a few hours of driving while in his intoxicated, broken state. He knew he would go to prison if he got caught driving with his current pending charges still on the line, so before even leaving the state of Texas, he put himself into a motel to go through withdrawal on his own.

I didn't learn about the volume of alcohol my son had been consuming daily until several months later. At his worst point, he could consume the equivalent volume of nearly ten bottles of wine in a day. I had been under the impression that it was significantly less than that. We had been through his withdrawals so many times by that point, it seemed like a predictable part of the process. Even with my medical education, I'm embarrassed to say I didn't fully understand the risks of what he did for three days alone in a motel room, risking seizures or sudden cardiac death. If we had understood the risks of withdrawal, we would have hospitalized him for the process.

He said he had to fill himself with as much Pedialyte as he could handle and just stay in a warm shower for as long as he was able to stand. He'd crawl from the bed to the shower and back to the bed, vomiting, sweating, and shaking for hours.

Even knowing he was alone and hurting, isolated in a motel room, I would waffle between feelings of terror and avoidance—telling myself at one minute that he'd be okay and the next, thinking he'd be better off dead so that he wouldn't suffocate under the debilitating awareness of suicidal depression. Then I'd realize less than a millisecond later that if I actually lost him, my devastation would swallow me whole. The brain battles its own World War, but no one ever wins, and the war never ends.

There I was, nearly ten long years into a death-defying addiction, and I still didn't fully grasp what withdrawal could do to him. I didn't understand when he was in solitary confinement, and I didn't comprehend how serious it was in the motel.

What was wrong with me? Was I avoiding the facts so that I could convince myself that it wasn't actually happening? Did my avoidance keep me in the dark to protect my fragility? He could have died in that hotel or that jail. The magnitude of that will haunt me for a lifetime. The grand lesson was to stop avoiding the truth that was laid bare right in front of me.

By the grace of God, Tyler survived three hellish days of withdrawal and got back on the road. He drove nearly twenty hours, sleeping in his vehicle halfway. He arrived a broken-down soul. He knew he had made a mistake and told us he didn't really have an explanation for his behavior. He said he felt things were actually going well before he left and that his relationship with us was good. He said he knew he was being impulsive even while doing it, but it was as if he didn't have control over that impulsivity—as if something else were controlling him. Maybe that's the definition of a hijacked brain.

Soon after his return, my son got a job and became curious about getting his own apartment to the point that we looked for some together. He agreed to start an antidepressant and to try *biofeedback*, which is a therapy that reinforces healthy brain function through operant conditioning or positive reinforcement. We even looked into *transcranial magnetic stimulation*, an even more intensive therapy, using electromagnetic induction.

He was on board, all the way up to the point when we noticed the slurred speech, the mood swings, and his lack of focus—meaning, he had started drinking once again and the hope of trying another therapy was gone. All along, we had been trying to help him treat the addiction without addressing the underlying mental health. When confronted with a breathalyzer test, he stormed out and was missing for three days.

This time, we had placed a tracker on his vehicle. I was prepared to go to him when he would call with his warning of wanting to die, but I had finally learned that I needed to let it play out until that call came. This is *the* hardest experience you will ever go through—the waiting, the fear, the unknown—as the loved one of an addict. It has no name, but some may compare it to torture. His intoxicated suicidal calls became more frequent, but I thoroughly understand now it was his way of calling for help.

Ultimately, the pain of waiting paid off. On day three, he called to tell me he couldn't handle it anymore, and he was going to AA. After the meeting, he called and asked if he was allowed to come back to the house just for the night and to get a shower. With caution, I agreed. Within a few hours of his arrival, the pain in his gut became unbearable, and he begged to be taken to the hospital.

This would be the first of three trips to the Emergency Room, but I was tone deaf to the severity of the physical effects playing out. It took us an hour to get to the hospital. At least half the time, he hung his head out of the window to prevent any potential vomit from invading my car. I'm not sure how you can have a level of awareness enough to avoid messing up someone's car after years of emotional damage, but here it was, and he remained consistently thoughtful throughout all those years.

At the ER, I told the registering nurse that my son was experiencing intractable vomiting due to alcohol abuse and asked the nurse point blank to please treat him with dignity. I guess I went in with the strong assumption that they would automatically give me the eye roll and throw any respect for an alcoholic out the window. After working in the ED and living through the nightmare that happened in Austin, Texas, we all had a heightened fear of mistreatment of addicted patients.

To my surprise, however, they helped us without hesitation. Later my son mentioned that a nurse had told him she formerly had a problem with opioids herself, so she completely understood his situation. Another nurse talked candidly with my son and told him he really should go to detox. My son agreed, and immediately after discharge, we drove him to the Wilmington Treatment Center.

I exhaled once again when he agreed to go. Each time I felt relieved and hopeful, but I was fearful change would not happen yet. Alex and I knew we would get a limited break from the chaos while Tyler was tucked away in a heavily guarded treatment facility, but we also knew that he would have to rebuild upon his release, and that was becoming its own trigger for relapse. We were learning the need for sobriety resources such as housing, jobs, counseling, and a local AA. We could only hope the treatment facility was geared toward transitional rehabilitation. Some facilities were better than others at this.

He did well overall at this particular treatment center and came home with renewed hope for maintaining his sobriety—always with the renewed hope. He moved in with one of his fellow rehab patients, and they became hard and fast friends. Initially, they were so good for one another and kept each other accountable. They maintained their friendship garnered through the rehab and attended AA and NA together for three straight months.

Tyler got a tree-cutting job from another sober friend, but several weeks into the job, his friend fell eighty feet out of a tree.

Miraculously, his friend did not sever his spinal cord as initially believed. He broke his vertebrae, hips, and legs and was ultimately transported to a major hospital in Georgia for patients with paraplegic and quadriplegic injuries. He was in recovery there for more than six months. This experience altered his ability to do the job, and the company suffered as a result of the accident. Tyler had to find other employment. The traumatic change started his usual nosedive into copious amounts of alcohol.

The friend who fell from the tree visited Alex and me. I'll never forget when he told me that he had encountered a lot of people over the years due to both his disease of addiction and his more recent recovery from the fall, but that Tyler stood out from them all. He said that Tyler was a uniquely special guy, and he was lucky to have met him.

As the months went on, the friends Tyler made in rehab and AA in Wilmington started falling off the sober train. One friend overdosed. Others started using again, which is not unusual, and his roommate followed suit. Tyler always seemed to follow in the footsteps of the people he loved the most. If they were sober, he was sober, and if they started using again, he seemed to find solace in using again as well. It was almost as if he had been given permission to drink again, and he took it. I was unaware of what was happening at the time because Tyler kept me in the dark; however, I remained chained to that ever-faithful hope.

All I knew was that I got three months of his sobriety, and this time, it included my birthday and Christmas. I was so happy during that time. He had really hit it off with a girl he met. Her name was Kate. He revealed that she was *the one* on October 26, 2020. I wrote down the date because I didn't want to forget it.

Tyler and Kate came to me bearing gifts on my birthday. The gifts were over the top and expensive. He shouldn't have spent all that money, I told him, but he said he had a lot of making up to do, so I just enjoyed the moment. His gifts were so thoughtful. He had been paying attention to details when I thought he hadn't. I loved everything he gave me, but I would have been just as happy with his visit alone. Kate brought me flowers—the first I'd ever received from one of his girlfriends—and she was as beautiful as the flowers. We got to know one another. It all seemed so normal.

A few weeks later, we enjoyed Christmas Day together. It was a bit different, and my radar wasn't fully operable. I was still riding high after that over-the-top birthday experience. He made some excuse about not being able to arrive until much later that day. I had bought breakfast sweet rolls for everyone with plans to open the Christmas gifts somewhat early that morning, like we used to do when Tyler was little. I called the late start a loss and didn't worry about it. He kept texting and making excuses about why they were still running late, but they eventually arrived around 2:00 p.m. I had learned a long time ago to pick my battles, and this wasn't one of them. I just let it go.

We had a good day. We opened gifts and ate our Christmas meal together. He went upstairs for a while, but I assumed he was just watching TV. They went home soon after dinner with very full bellies and smiles on their faces. I felt good and normal and relieved. Hope was trying to creep in. I went to bed and slept well that night. Tyler and I texted and talked by phone a few times over the next few weeks, but the signs began to seep in, and I later learned he had been drinking on Christmas Day and from then on.

Several weeks into January 2021, after about a month of sitting back and trying desperately to let natural consequences occur, I called my son and asked if he would meet me for brunch. I had a few items for him, and I wanted to see him in the flesh. I wasn't expecting to see what I actually saw. He arrived looking completely broken, weak, and defeated. He looked a lot older than his years.

Tyler's face was swollen, and even with the wind as strong as it was that day, I could smell the overwhelming stench of alcohol coming from his pores. I was thankful for the mandatory use of masks due to the pandemic, not just for me, but for everyone we walked by. We paid the cashier, and I followed my son to a table in the back, away from others. I was bowled over by the smell trailing behind him in a wave so thick I was surprised it wasn't visible. My heart sank to a low point I had become quite familiar with.

We sat at a high-top and made small talk. I presented a gift for him from his grandmother. She had sent it to our house right after Christmas, and this was the first time I had seen Tyler since then. I had no idea what the gift was but assumed it would be useful because she always knew what he needed. I never expected to see what it was or how he would react.

He opened the gift to find his grandfather's dog tags. He looked up with huge tears in his eyes and we both immediately started crying. His grandpa, my father, always had this mysterious attachment with Tyler. Because of divorce, my dad wasn't in my life as much and consequently, not in Tyler's either, but they were always somehow very connected.

After catching his composure somewhat, he said, "It's so hard to explain, but even though I didn't know Grandpa that well, I have always felt so close to him, like he's watching out for me."

Through my tears, I said I had always felt the same way.

He read the note from his Grandma Carol expressing how much love she had for him, but she also made the comment that not all wars are fought on the battlefield. It was truly a beautiful exchange between Tyler and me. He immediately put the dog tags around his neck and said he refused to ever take them off. He wears them to this day.

I looked across the table at my son with agony in my heart. I said, "I will take you back to detox or rehab if you want me to."

For the first time, he simply nodded as if to say: *I surrender*. We were both surrendering at this point. We finished what we could of our meal. After such a heavy emotional experience, most of what we had ordered remained on the plates untouched.

At home later, I made a few phone calls and located a rehabilitation facility that met our needs in terms of proximity, cost, and approach, or so I thought.

CHAPTER 9

A WELL-WORN PATH

Addiction is the only disease that tells you you're not sick.
~ Unknown

Let's say you decide to go for a walk in a wooded park. It would make sense that when you arrive, you find a path cleared of debris, sticks, weeds, and fallen trees. You walk where so many before you have walked and cleared the way to hike in the woods.

Similarly, after repeatedly subjecting the brain to an addictive substance, a clean, cleared neural pathway is created. You can learn to create a new path by clearing away all the brush and fallen branches by stopping the use of your drug of choice, but it will always be easier to return to the habitually cleared path when it comes to smoking cigarettes, gambling, overeating, or using cocaine, for example. Just like a bowling ball tends to fall into the groove of the side gutter—or at least it does it my case—the brain's response in active addiction will slide most easily into the well-worn neural pathway. And that addiction groove, made in the matrix of our brains, stays there for a lifetime. The hope is that eventually the habituated path will be completely covered by debris while the new clean path has been created.

Visual comparisons can help simplify this disease and assist in the understanding, in most cases, the irreversible effects on the brain.

However, there are multiple influences that are all chapters in a massive novel of disease interpretation, such as:

- Genetics
- Environmental factors
- Reward dysregulation
- Personality traits
- Neurotransmission of feel-good chemical messengers

Simplified, substance use disorder is multifactorial. It becomes important to understand the physiology of this disease to comprehend and diffuse the breadth of emotions, such as anger and resentment, you can misdirect toward your loved one. Ideally, we learn that it is hard to dislike someone when we know they have an all-consuming disease they never asked for.

Fortunately, addiction has been studied and written about extensively by knowledgeable experts. They have provided a breadth of information to learn from. For these purposes, I simply want to provide the superficial understanding needed to make it through this complex experience you may be struggling to comprehend about your loved one.

When I talk to my patients, I provide only the details they want to learn about. I try to keep it as straightforward as possible. That is the same thing I want to do here for you, but as I said, there are thousands of available resources if you're ready to dive deeper.

Genetics

From the moment of conception, my son, like many others, had nearly every probability of acquiring the disease of addiction based on his genetic vulnerability alone. It is well understood that if Mom and Dad both have green eyes, there is a very high likelihood that their offspring will also have green eyes. In the same way, the genetic acquisition of addiction has also become much better understood. Simply put, if there is a history of substance abuse in your family, there can be a higher probability—most studies suggest at least a 50 percent increased risk—that your child will have addictive tendencies.

Beyond the *nature versus nurture* debate, there is further genetic research in yet another layer, called *epigenetics*. This examines heritable characteristics—how the gene is ultimately expressed—that result not from alteration in the DNA sequence, but from external or environmental factors. In the same way high blood pressure is a consequence of both your genetics and your lifestyle, addiction is about so much more than your DNA alone.

The good news is that a heritable vulnerability to addiction does not mean substance abuse is cemented in, but it is relevant information for future generations. My son's father and his paternal grandfather are both predisposed to substance use disorder. Members of my family who passed away before I was born carried the disease of alcoholism. My son's genetic coding existed long before he was even thought of, and he certainly has epigenetic factors that have contributed to his substance abuse.

To sum it up, having substance use disorder may be highly suggestive of having the genetic coding in your family tree, but having the genetic coding does not necessarily mean you will have substance use disorder. With all that we've learned, I can't help but worry about what my potential grandchildren would be up against.

It's not critical to know about the genetic factors when trying to help your loved one in active addiction, but it may be important to know the impact the genetic mapping has in your family. Interestingly, there has been research on an addiction vaccine since the 1970s. If that actually came to pass, we would be able to vaccinate the children of individuals with alcohol use disorder to help prevent further suffering.

Environmental Factors

I still believe that some simplified explanations of causality can be helpful in alleviating misperceptions, especially when you're trying to help extended family understand what is really happening. Placing an individual with the genetic makeup for addiction potential in the wrong environment may contribute to substance use disorder. A person's environment can include their home, school, work, social events, and peer groups. If your loved one's environment is one in which drugs or alcohol are available and widely accepted, it can have a strong effect on their potential for abuse and addiction. I don't think I'm sharing any earth-shattering new information; rather, I'm supplying possible variables that are pieces of a puzzle.

Our home did not support regular use of alcohol, nor did we use it as a coping mechanism at any time. We did have alcohol in our home when our son was growing up in a new neighborhood, school, and peer group. Looking back now, would it have made any difference if it had never been there?

My son *found God in a bottle*, as he called it, when he would visit his father and found it was easy to use any amount he wanted in that environment. We were completely left in the dark about his newfound hideaway at his dad's house. It honestly never occurred to me to remind his father that his son shouldn't drink alcohol at the age of twelve. I don't think Tyler's dad knew the extent of his son's drinking in his home, but Tyler's dad, who would often be under the influence of alcohol himself, will admit he was rarely tuned in when he should have been.

Moving to a new neighborhood and school right at the time of identity formation proved to be a mistake. People have to do it all the time when parents take a new job, or the military transfers a parent to a new base or post. Many of us get through it, but everyone is different, and for my son, it overwhelmed his primed system.

The young tweens in his new environment were mostly cruel, and this wasn't old-time locker-room bullying; the internet is a powerful tool. He was an outsider, and they made him aware of that every day. To make matters more difficult, Tyler was a nonconformist in a small conformist town. He was left out when all he wanted to do was fit in, as we all want. The effects of bullying and meanness can have long-lasting, even lifelong, consequences, and in my son's case, they have been. I don't lay blame solely on the backs of those young individuals, but they were certainly a part of the compounding effects of my son's story.

The online world may be the worst environment of all. The social media effect has played a part in demolishing our sense of well-being and replaced it with self-doubt, loneliness, and insecurity, in many cases. I just have to wonder whether my son would be dealing with the severity of his disease if he had grown up before the internet. The predator and the bullies in my son's story all thrived there.

Neurotransmission and Reward Dysregulation

In trying to make sense of the baffling neuroscience behind addiction, one thing I read in the book *Never Enough*, by Judith Grisel, made more of an impact on my understanding of my son's addiction than almost anything else. She looked specifically at endorphins, which are hormones secreted in the brain and nervous system that activate the body's opiate receptors, relieving pain. After analyzing studies of more specific effects of beta-endorphins in addiction, and specifically in alcohol addiction, she wrote of them, "Dr. Gianoulakis and her colleagues showed that high-risk individuals have about half as much beta-endorphin in their blood as those at low genetic risk; Jan Froehlich and her colleagues then showed these levels come largely from our parents" (2019). *Beta-endorphin* is an endorphin produced in the pituitary gland that is a powerful pain suppressor—it can inhibit communication of pain signals and may also produce a feeling of euphoria very similar to that produced by other opioids.

She went on to write:

> But most interesting to me was the fact that the alcohol was able to remedy this natural deficit especially in those who inherit a high risk for excessive drinking, and at higher doses, produce a surfeit of the peptide. Because beta-endorphin contributes to a sense of well-being by soothing stress and facilitating social affiliation, those of us with naturally low levels may experience less sense of safety and connection even as children on a day-to-day basis, that is until John Barleycorn is invited to the party! Data such as these suggest that some of us are especially likely to find alcohol reinforcing because we can use it to medicate an innate opioid deficiency.

She then wrote the very words I've heard my son use when describing how he felt most of the time: "Perhaps the 'hole in my soul'

I felt finally filled in my friend's basement was nothing more than a flood of endorphins at last, quenching destitute receptors." *Bingo!* In Tyler's case, that made more sense than any other explanation available.

I also began to recognize the patterns of use my son developed. It took years for my eyes to open to the pattern he had been forming. I later equated his addiction relapses to the likes of a PTSD response. A continuous loop of brain-trained pacification is what I witnessed. When fireworks or gunshots go off, those with PTSD can sometimes have a warzone, fox-hole-type response and hunker down to avoid the danger. When those with substance use disorder experience triggers—sights, sounds, smells, or events that can elicit substance use—they also find what helps to soothe the brain and avoid pain or danger. It becomes second nature to self-medicate when anxiety becomes too overwhelming for the system. It becomes their only coping skill, and there's a whole cascade of neurotransmission that's occurring behind the curtain.

To put it a bit more plainly, drugs and alcohol affect the dopamine centers of your brain, the *feel-good* areas also known as your *reward pathway*, which can activate opioid receptors and dopamine release. Dopamine is involved with motivation, memory, reward, and attention. When it's released, it creates feelings and memories of pleasure, which motivate you to repeat a specific behavior. And repeat, and repeat, and repeat.

Drugs like heroin, fentanyl, OxyContin, morphine, and alcohol rewire your brain with continued use. Every time you provide the brain with an outside source, such as an addictive substance, you get an excessive dopamine spike. It feels not just *good*, but earth-shatteringly good. Normal pleasurable experiences can no longer cause the release of mountains of dopamine your brain has become accustomed to, leading to cravings to re-create the level of pleasure you reflexively desire.

Driving a fast car on a racetrack under normal circumstances, for example, will release a level of dopamine that feels good and will likely make you want to do it more. However, when an addict drives fast in that same car, they likely won't experience the same amount of pleasure because their brain has become quite accustomed to extreme levels of dopamine release caused by using their drug of choice. After a while, a person won't feel normal *without* taking these drugs. Rather than using their drug of choice for its enjoyable effects, your loved one will over-satiate their addiction to keep from feeling bad.

Addiction isn't a matter of wanting to feel good; it becomes a desperate attempt to feel normal. Resetting the natural dopamine release in addiction after a person stops using is variable dependent, but chronic use can require months to years for the brain to completely recuperate, although some measurable healing can start in as early as two to four weeks, so there is hope.

Personality Traits
Theories of addiction pivoting on personality are also complex. A valid examination of *affective states*, or personality traits or modes of thinking, will help to further break down the preconceived ideas of moral failing. Put simply, it means people with mood disorders are at increased risk of substance use disorder.

Mood disorders can include:
- Major depressive disorder
- Generalized anxiety disorder

- Bipolar disorder
- Attention deficit/hyperactivity disorder—ADD and ADHD
- PTSD
- Schizophrenia

Again, these may not be relevant when helping someone in active addiction, but my goal here is to help you with the global understanding of substance use disorder and to diffuse the frustration and resentment that builds over the years. After all, it is said, holding on to resentments is like drinking poison and expecting the other person to die.

As a medical professional, it's my job to understand the physiological processes of addiction, but as a guilt-ridden mom, I was a bottomless chasm when it became an obsession to understand the underlying mechanisms of addiction. I feel like I went on some literary quest to get to the core of why my son was given this particular burden. I devoured book after book. His disease became an enigma. I set out to crack this impossible puzzle all on my own. This is how over-the-top people can become when their loved one has substance use disorder. Thankfully, many scientists are working tirelessly toward answering these same questions, so loved ones and family members can allow their brains to rest. Maybe it's time to let the highly educated and more-than-qualified medical practitioners, scientists, and researchers find the answers we all have been looking for.

I hoped for a cure to be found in my son's lifetime, and I still do; however, I hadn't quite recognized I needed the same cure, so my own addiction to him could find its own remission.

The problem was, I had to fully accept that I couldn't cure his disease. The saying in Al-Anon, *You didn't cause it, you can't control it, and you can't cure it* was laid bare before my eyes.

Again, I thought: *What do they know? Not only* can *I do it; I have to!*

Reality check—Nope! I alone cannot, and no one else has been able to either. So where has this overinflated sense of self or ability come from? The same place it comes from in all of us: from a limitless love for our children. I wanted and needed answers more than my son did. I cared more about the answer than he ever did about the question.

Maybe with this disease, finding the why at some point should stop taking priority. One mother told me her daughter was diagnosed with lung cancer when she was fourteen.

The mother went on the same relentless crusade to find the answer to why until one day a nurse said, "There may not be a reason, but right now, the point is to stop looking back for answers and to start looking forward to the life your daughter has." Several years later, her daughter became an addict, and once again, a mom was lost, with no reasonable answers to the why of it all.

Knowledge is power; but I should add, knowledge in moderation, like everything else, is very helpful. Consuming nothing but information about your loved one's disease can become crippling. That is why I tried to present concise information without going into the abyss and confusing the point. The point is your survival in the midst of their addiction.

CHAPTER 10

GUT INSTINCTS

You know the truth by the way it feels.
~ Unknown

The rehab facility in South Carolina had recently started a separate detox program in early 2021. I was so thankful and asked if I could bring my son there that Sunday, which was the next day. They said he needed to be there by 1:00 p.m. in order to get him admitted. I probably don't have to tell you that when an addict is in withdrawal, their willingness to go to rehab or detox is not, and never will be, on a schedule—most detox facilities are open for 24-hour admissions—but I accepted their proposal under the strained circumstances.

Knowing it would be a four- to five-hour drive, I told my son over the phone I would have to pick him up by 8:00 a.m. He said he couldn't do it—his girlfriend would be going back to work, and it was the last day for over a month that he would see her. Always the excuses.

Tyler explained that when he woke up in the mornings, it took several hours just to get past the most dreaded experience of his day. He described it as *not wanting to be alive* until he had enough alcohol in his system that he felt relatively normal and functional. This was something I had no understanding of. I felt sympathy, but I simply could not relate, and of course, you want to be able to understand where your child is coming from when they are hurting so deeply.

I told him I could arrange for a 2:00 p.m. arrival at the facility, and if we didn't make any stops, we could leave at 10:00 a.m. He agreed, and I was thankful and momentarily relieved. I called the rehab center and explained the situation, but right then and there they said no; they were terribly sorry, but they could not accommodate the request under any circumstances.

That should have been a huge red flag, but desperate times catapulted me into desperate measures. I agreed to have him there by 1:00 that Monday; however, this gave him more time to fill his gut with unimaginable quantities of alcohol. I made every effort to get him there as early as I could that morning.

My son walked out of his apartment with a broken plastic laundry basket filled with a few socks, T-shirts, pairs of underwear, and sweats. None of it appeared clean. On top of the heap of clothes was a half-emptied magnum of cheap white wine.

"What do you think you're going to do with that?" I asked.

He said it was the only way he could get down to rehab, since the drive would take several hours. I knew trying to haggle with someone under the influence was worse than trying to take away a sippy cup from a three-year-old, so I did not battle him over the bottle. He climbed in, and we got through the first hour of the drive without any serious complications. The last three were a terrorizing hellish experience I wouldn't wish on my worst enemy. I should never have done the drive with my son on my own.

As Tyler's alcohol level rose in his blood, so did his emotional instability. He asked to play music from his iPhone. I reluctantly agreed just trying to placate him any way I could think to do so. He fumbled terribly trying to set up his Bluetooth to work through my vehicle. He was crying and frustrated because he couldn't get his hands to function normally due to his intoxication.

I was repeating to myself: *Just get there, just get there*, in my head. He would roll down the window and put up his middle finger for no reason or reach over and lay on my horn while I was driving more than 80 miles per hour.

It was a completely volatile situation. He spilled wine all over the floor and on his pants multiple times while attempting to pour it into a tumbler. He eventually started screaming the obviously emotional lyrics and looking at me with pure agony in his eyes, trying desperately to will me to understand what he was actually feeling.

At one point he put his hand on my knee when he saw I was crying too. This is something he had never done before. I knew it came out of the vulnerable place that only alcohol permitted for him. He could communicate lovingly with me when the alcohol gave him the ability to let his guard down. A moment that gave him an ounce of peace was so very painful for me.

He asked me many times to pull over, so he could pee. When we would stop, I would pour out just enough of the wine onto the ground for him not to notice. We got to a point when he said he couldn't hold it anymore. I pulled into the back of a gas station. Initially, he got out and fumbled with his zipper. I grabbed the bottle and put the whole thing right outside my driver's door.

He was too intoxicated to notice. I could see how much he was struggling on the other side of the car. I got out and held him up while he tried to urinate. He got pee all down the front of his wine-soaked pants. It was such a filthy mess, and when I looked up there were two people watching us. I quickly got him in the car, and we drove away, leaving the wine bottle and those two voyeurs in our rearview mirror. We still had more than an hour before we would arrive for detox.

It didn't get much better, but he calmed down slightly. When we finally turned down the gravel road leading to the facility, I pulled over to the side. With my voice quivering, I asked God to watch over Tyler during this stay at rehab and to bring the right people along his path so that he could recover. I asked that the craving for alcohol and any other substance be removed from him for good. I thanked God for having another day with my son and said amen. Tyler didn't say anything, and we just drove up to the compound.

Several people were outside playing basketball when we arrived. My son made some alcohol-influenced comment about them and said, "I don't want to see people with their bullshit sobriety. It's all so fake." Tyler called and cried to his girlfriend one last time, then stumbled out of the passenger's seat. We walked in, and my son immediately turned up his defensive and embarrassing argumentative behavior fueled by the alcohol.

Initially he argued with the admission counselor when she told him that his cigarettes and vape products were not allowed during detox. He threw a temper tantrum and threw himself down on the ground saying he was going to leave. The counselor negotiated with him, and eventually, he gave up his power struggle with her.

I said to the admissions counselor, "Well, this is embarrassing, but I promise he'll be your best friend by the time he leaves here."

We were in a small, brown office with a standard-issue desk and two chairs. They told us they needed to do Tyler's intake and that a nurse would be on his way. Tyler was slumped over and appeared barely alive in the corner chair. He looked like he had just been through ten rounds of a knockout fight. I *felt* like I had. Eventually, a new intake nurse arrived. I asked if I should step out during this part of the interview, but they said it wasn't necessary. I questioned that in my head but also knew the state my son was in and didn't necessarily want to leave him just yet.

Tyler, still with piss and wine all over his dirty clothes, was barely able to breathe, let alone supply critical information. I tried to fill in the blanks where I could, and he answered when he could. There was one particular question I was not prepared for. The new nurse asked Tyler if he had ever exchanged sex for drugs or alcohol in the past. Without hesitation, he said yes. The punch in my gut was immediate and intense. I acted normal on the outside, like I already knew this information, but I was screaming on the inside. *Did anyone else just hear what my son said?* I wanted to scream out loud: *Does he realize I'm standing right here? Does anyone realize I'm standing here? Am I ever going to wake up from this nightmare? God, can you seriously hear me?!*

I don't think the nurse's question was supposed to be asked in front of me. I would have been better off never knowing that part of his past. I'm not angry that I know, but I'm angry they didn't consider whether or not he wanted me to know. It made me realize how far he went simply because, as he always had, he felt it is what he thought he deserved.

I remain baffled by this self-sabotaging internal storm that he has tried to deal with most of his life and by his disconnection from the love I had for him. But I also know now that his actions had nothing to do with me or how much I loved him. The information and the secrets you learn over time can be overwhelming. I'm not sure what a mother is supposed to do with the amount of information put into her consciousness.

I had no clue there was so much worse to come.

Here's my takeaway: Don't go into your loved one's intake at any facility with them. There are some things better left unknown.

The questioning seemed to take forever, and I couldn't exactly understand the purpose of a full intake when the patient is in this particular state. They finally started asking questions about physical signs and symptoms. They asked if he recently had dark, tarry stools, which can be a sign of potential internal bleeding. He said yes, and they stopped everything right then and there. They told me I had to take him to the hospital and that it was unsafe to have him stay if he had an active bleed. They were right to send us to the hospital, but they didn't realize they were sending us into the pandemic abyss. And they sent me without a safety net.

CHAPTER 11

RAISING THE WHITE FLAG

*When we are no longer able to change a situation . . .
we are challenged to change ourselves.*
~ Victor E. Frankl
Man's Search for Meaning

When we arrived at the hospital, the waiting room was completely full, likely because of Covid or maybe because of something else. My focus was elsewhere. I helped Tyler check in, and for the second time, I asked staff for their mercy and respect when treating my son. As the day was turning into night several hours later, I called Alex and explained I would likely not make it home that night.

We were getting to a point when my son's blood alcohol content was dipping to a degree of noticeable distress. He kept saying he needed some alcohol to get through this ordeal and avoid going into withdrawal. He was rocking back and forth, holding his arms over his stomach and moaning in pain. It was a physical pain that was so foreign to me, but as a mother I could actually feel it. Seeing my child hurting was debilitating, but knowing the mental pain he was struggling with was too much to bear. I was the only one who knew of that pain, and there was still so much more to be revealed.

As we waited, I sat in crushing fear, worrying whether he'd dart out the door into the unknown or stay to be treated. He had walked away before, actually ran, when we and others had tried to get him to detox, so my fear was unrelenting. I distracted him and put it off as long as I possibly could, but after at least four hours of waiting, I did the worst thing a mother could find herself doing: I left him so I could purchase the very poison for which he was being treated. It was my only bargaining chip, but it was excruciatingly painful for me. I went to a gas station, bought the wine and some chips and cried all the way back to the hospital. Someone had to stay in case he was called, and he was willing to do that if I would do my part of the bargain.

As soon as I got there, he rushed out to the car and drank half the bottle. I told him I would only go once, so he needed to make it last. You'll honestly say anything in desperate situations, I've discovered. About once every hour, I would ask when he might be called back. I was becoming completely unhinged and nearly hysterical after six hours of waiting.

Around this time, Tyler collapsed into my arms in total distress. He was quietly crying into my lap, and I was rubbing his back. He was in a lot of pain from a condition we were soon to learn more about. Eventually a nurse came and talked to me because someone noticed I was about to have my own panic attack. She apologized and said they were intubating Covid patients left and right, and multiple codes were being called at the same time. She said there were no beds available in the ED and the only place they could put Tyler was in the hallway.

I said, "You can put him anywhere because watching over him and worrying that at any second, he is going to leave into this unknown city in the darkness is about to make me lose it."

It took another hour, but someone came and drew his blood. Awhile later, they pulled us from the waiting room and put us in a hallway away from the other patients. She told us he most likely had pancreatitis based on the labs they got when he arrived, and they needed to get some imaging. He would be put in a bed in the hall very soon. She explained he would need to be admitted that night, so I might as well go home and get some rest. She also said that he typically would have been considered high acuity and, in a typical situation, would have been a top-priority triage patient.

Covid created his significant delay in care. Covid made me buy my son alcohol so that I could keep him there. I would blame anything I could for our suffering by this time. I felt so angry and frustrated, and now, without food or clothes—let alone a toothbrush—I needed to check into a hotel and stay the night. I walked out of the hospital in a fugue state, completely bewildered and exhausted. I managed to buy a few necessities from a drugstore and found a hotel nearby.

I finally lay my head down, and right then, my son called. He said he was going to walk out of the hospital because no one had even seen him yet. This was eleven hours after our arrival. I knew he had to be dealing with severe cravings by this point. I tried negotiating with him. I told him someone would be there soon, and then I promised to call the nurses' station and ask what was happening. Almost the same time I called, someone finally went to see him, and they gave him his saving grace—Ativan, a sedative that can help reduce anxiety, prevent seizures, and calm the nervous system. This enabled both of us to get some sleep.

I went to the hospital bright and early the next morning. He was legitimately scared of his diagnosis. Tyler was groggy and grouchy, a disposition I was used to, but I sat with him for as long as I was allowed.

The hospitalist came in and minimized his condition. This frustrated me because I felt Tyler needed to hear from a professional how he was damaging his body, how he was going to kill himself if he kept up the level of drinking he had become accustomed to. Instead she suggested he might be discharged. I called the rehab facility and said we may be back there soon. I think they were afraid to deal with someone in his condition and told me they couldn't take him again, because it was after 1:00 p.m.

At this point, I broke down. I was in an unknown city, I was hungry and sleep deprived, I had checked out of my hotel, I had been wearing the same clothes since we arrived, and they were telling me they couldn't take him?

"What am I supposed to do? How am I supposed to manage an addict in withdrawal in a hotel by myself? How could you do this to me?" I asked. But why wasn't I asking how Tyler could do this to me? Because there was never a time I felt he was doing anything *to me*—I knew this was what he was doing to himself, and I was just the collateral damage.

I called the administrator of the rehab facility to ask if there was any way the hospital could find a reason for him to stay another night until he could go to the rehab facility. After an hour of biting my nails and feeling confused and angry, I received word Tyler would be at the hospital for another night. I felt like I had been in a boxing ring for days at this point. The beating I took might as well have been physical because I felt every aching bone and muscle in my body.

When I went to breakfast the next morning, the woman serving looked at me and asked if I was okay.

"Not really," I said, and tears welled up in my eyes.

She looked at me and said, "It's gonna be okay. I'll pray for you." What innocent sweetness from a pure stranger! There was still good in the world.

I arrived at Tyler's room and sat watching television while he slept. It was during a very tumultuous time in our country, and yet, I was so removed, I could have been anywhere in the world right then. I felt so empty and drained.

I was growing furious with my son. I was angry that he didn't recognize all I had given up just to be sitting there with him for three days. I was angry he had gotten to the point of needing to be hospitalized. I was angry for being angry. Depression and rage became my existence. I finally arrived at the destination of hopelessness and despair. I gave up and tried to raise a white flag that nobody could see. I said the words out loud to my husband that I had officially lost all hope. I became unrecognizable to myself.

Tyler was finally discharged, and when we arrived back at the facility, he was much calmer and resigned. I had hoped he was fully ready to surrender yet again, but it wasn't meant to happen here. After one week in detox and two weeks in recovery, he called his girlfriend to pick him up, and she did. He left early and started drinking again within three days. There had to be some revelation that occurred because this was when Tyler dropped the bomb into our life about his real experience ten years before.

What he confided forced me to think about everything completely differently. A veil had been lifted, and what was under it was the darkest part of human existence you'd never want to know about.

CHAPTER 12

DAMAGED SOUL

In some ways, it's my rage that keeps me going.
~ Etta James

On a random weekday in 2021, I was FaceTiming with Tyler. He had been living with his girlfriend, Kate, and found himself at home after he lost another job. He was desperately trying to make small talk when I noticed he was having a hard time. He had started crying, and I could see he was fidgeting with the knife he was using to cut up some vegetables. He was also intoxicated. The next moment, as if out of nowhere, he cried out, "Mom—I was raped!"

He held on to the counter in his kitchen as if the universe were going to suck him into a black hole right then from the force of releasing the darkest part of his soul. It was an explosive release of agony after a decade of attempting to suppress it all with alcohol.

Tyler used the word *rape*, not assaulted, not abused, but rape—one of the vilest words in the English language. Tears of misplaced shame streamed down his face as he convulsed in sobs. The world turned instantly dark. Ten long years of pain exploded right in front of me. All the air was pulled from my lungs. I now understood trauma had been a part of the picture all along. Rage washed over me. The only thing I remember after that moment was being on my knees, crying.

My son was the target of an online predator who also happened to be a major university football coach. This was before the great media blitz to warn parents of the potential yet real dangers lurking on their child's computer. The monsters you've heard about are real. Here was a self-conscious teenager struggling with his self-esteem and an already brewing alcohol appreciation. He was an ideal target, and apparently, I was a distracted parent.

I believe now that for all those years my son had been in a soundproof box, screaming and punching the walls right in front of our eyes, blood streaming from his knuckles, and we were unable to see or hear him. We were laughing and carrying on with life as if it all were somehow normal. Life played this evil trick on him, and on all of us really.

I tried to go back to 2012 in my mind a million times to see what I had missed. I don't know if I've erased any uncomfortable memories from that time or if he was a master of disguise and never showed any overt signs of being assaulted. Regardless, I feel as if I've failed him.

I thought maybe he decided to tell me when he did because he was ready for it all to be over and he didn't want me to carry the guilt of thinking I had done something wrong for the rest of my life, which of course I had been thinking. I also fantasized that it would be some catalyst for his ultimate reckoning, and he would get the help he needed and be healthy once again. Renewed, reborn, resurrected is all that I ever prayed for.

My son and I both have a passion for film and photography, but we never saw the world through the same lens. The morning before he told me what happened to him, we had gone to breakfast, and I had assumed, as usual, that he would be sober. He drove to meet me, so of course, he wouldn't have had anything to drink, right? Except as soon as he arrived, I knew, and he knew I knew, so we had that uncomfortable interaction that alcoholics and nonalcoholics have. I felt compelled to get some food, water, and coffee into him, even though I was angry. I was still in the dark about his reality, and I couldn't reconcile his decisions with life. Even though I tried to communicate my frustrations in a productive way, he would inevitably shut me down.

That morning, Tyler said, "You know, Mom, the world is a really dark place, and bad things happen all the time."

"Well you're right," I immediately said, with total lack of awareness, "But it's all in how you choose to look at it." I claimed a foolish optimism and saw the good in the universe even as it was falling down around me. After he revealed his truth, I saw something more. I wasn't going to let darkness in, but I was going to fight the evil in front of me.

I'm not really sure how you recover from knowing your child has been raped or that your child's innocence has been taken away by an evil force you're not allowed to kill. We all worked on our recovery independently and daily, and that will likely be true for the remainder of our lives to some degree. I pray that we will one day know all the pertinent information to charge the perpetrator for his crime. No evil goes unpunished in my just world. But my most earnest prayer is for the recovery of my son's joy—that he may see beauty in the universe once again.

Tyler often said, "I didn't ask to be born, and I didn't ask for this disease, and I don't want it." There's so much validity to that. He didn't ask to be born. I made that decision. I made it not knowing what he would be up against. But of course, that can be said for any life. We all face challenges and burdens, some more than others, and some can be dealt with better than others. There are just no guarantees.

I finally understand why he said those comments in the first place. As excruciating as it has all been, there has been some healing. Just knowing what happened to him helps me understand his choices. Some people self-harm by cutting themselves. He routinely self-harmed on a much larger scale: exchanging his body for harmful substances, going to jail, drinking to the point of organ damage. These are grander forms of self-harm, but so many individuals still see it as the user's moral failings.

Tyler came into this world a happy and grateful soul. We both did. I have no idea how that happens—why some are born with an irritable, frustrated existence and others with mere contentedness. But another soul came along, a discontented one, and tried to steal what we were born with. I think of the terror my son must have felt because of that monster. All I know is that he was victimized, drugged, and raped. My mind is left to fill in the blanks.

Tyler still struggles with blaming himself for what happened, as a lot of victims of rape do. He believes he should have been able to fight and get out of the situation. He never understood why he couldn't, even though the experts understand.

In multiple AA meetings and rehab group settings, Tyler had screamed out what had happened to him. He had revealed the assault to his sponsors, counselors, and a few close friends. It wasn't until he told me, his stepdad, and his girlfriend that he was able to start healing, although he had yet to tell his dad, and that would not be easy for him. He needed to know the people closest to him would still love him, despite what had happened. As his mother, I feel so much pain with this knowledge. How do I ever take away what Tyler has had to carry with him all these years? How do you make sure your child knows how much of your own soul they are?

CHAPTER 13

A LESSON IN TRAUMA

One day you will tell your story of how you overcame what you went through, and it will be someone else's survival guide.
~ often attributed to Brené Brown

When we talk about trauma, it is most commonly in reference to the individual in whom the trauma has occurred—as it should be. But how do we overcome the trauma that happened to someone we love? How do I remove the nightmares and visions I now have of what I believed happened to one of the most important people in my life, the one I was put here to protect? This book was born out of the hope that someone else can be saved as a result of speaking out.

First, I had to understand the effects of trauma. What were we really dealing with psychologically, physically, and emotionally? I had to methodically read and comprehend the psychology in order to help myself, and maybe my son, in the process. I learned a lot in my research on trauma, and it helped provide the global understanding I was searching for. The question of why, however, will never be answered, and giving up on asking that question is hard. Instead of looking for answers, I found a way to search for solutions because that's all I had in my control.

With all the knowledge and solution searching in the world, I still struggled to accept that evil lurks in plain sight. In *What Happened to You?* by Dr. Bruce Perry and Oprah Winfrey, I read something that finally made more sense than anything else had. It gave me clarity in reference to my own trauma:

> Often when a traumatic event takes place, it is so threatening and so far outside our usual experience that it doesn't fit our working model of the world. Our mind is always working to preserve the worldview that was created early in our lives. *People are good. Parents are here to protect us. Schools are safe.* The mind wants to see what we believe, so it clings to things that support those beliefs—that worldview—and ignores things that don't. But trauma shatters this inner landscape. Your worldviews are broken to pieces (2021).

My worldview has definitely been shattered, yet not destroyed. I am a survivor and so is my son. The predator is the one who lives in the dark, not us. He is the one who must hide while we live in the openness that is life. Well, that is, at least I do. My son is still working to rebuild his freedom.

Secondly, I learned how far from isolated my son's experience was. Trauma, especially sexually based traumas, are far more dispersed than I would ever want to accept. In *Waking the Tiger: Healing Trauma*, Peter A. Levine outlines that more than 40 percent of a thousand men and women studied had experienced some kind of traumatic event. Of those traumas, most were rapes or physical assaults, witnessing the death or injury of another person, or being in a serious accident. He also shared that between 75 million and 100 million Americans have experienced childhood sexual trauma and physical abuse.

Of the lasting effects of such experiences, he writes:

> Unresolved trauma can keep us excessively cautious and inhibited or lead us around in ever-tightening circles of dangerous reenactment, victimization, and unwise exposure to danger. We become the perpetual victims or therapy clients. Trauma can destroy the quality of our relationships and distort sexual experiences. When we do not resolve our traumas, we feel that we have failed, or that we have been betrayed by those we chose to help us (1997).

These numbers turned my understanding of trauma on its head. This information helped me understand how this trauma had such a profound effect on my son. Tyler had every imaginable expression of unhealed trauma.

It's a long list but reads like this:
- Lacking sense of self-worth
- Maintaining codependency in relationships
- Fearing abandonment
- Putting his needs aside for other people
- Craving external validation
- Feeling innately ashamed
- Not being able to tolerate conflict
- Fearing what might happen next
- Resisting positive change

- Tolerating abusive behaviors from others
- Difficulty standing up for himself and asserting boundaries
- Being overly agreeable

In addition, these symptoms might manifest for some people:
- Flashbacks
- Anxiety
- Panic attacks
- Insomnia
- Nightmares
- Depression
- Chronic body aches and pains from unknown sources
- Destructive behaviors

My son has experienced every one of these symptoms over the years. He often tried to express that he felt like he was going crazy or like he could have a mental breakdown at any moment, but I missed the signs that he had been through a trauma, even as it was presented directly in my face.

A particularly interesting fact I discovered when investigating the effects of trauma was how traumatized individuals can turn an intense aggression inward on themselves rather than allow it external expression. I equated that to the self-harm my son engaged in. The inward aggression was also expressed through years of my son having unimaginable nightmares. He never really told me what they were about because he said they were too horrible to reveal, but he would have them regularly for more than ten years.

It is also well known that drugs and alcohol can be used to escape these symptoms:

> *Many* traumatized people feel that they live in a personal hell in which no other human could possibly share. The result, sadly, is that many traumatized victims become riddled with fear and anxiety and are never fully able to feel at home with themselves or in the world (Levine 1997).

And what about our society's response to handling trauma?

I have this insatiable urge to ask that officer who took my son to jail instead of a mental health facility whether, if he had known my son had been abused by a university football coach, would the officer have approached the situation the same way? Or better yet—if it were his own child, how would he want them to be treated in the same situation?

How can we ever know what has happened to someone else? We simply cannot, so start from a place of understanding, not judgment.

An excerpt of my son's journal he shared with me:

> As we walk past people on the street or look at someone across the room at a quiet coffee shop, we have to make a conscious effort to simply understand that there is an entire universe in that one soul. We make a host of assumptions instead of leading with compassion. Every single human has a story. Every one of us.

CHAPTER 14

CRISIS INTERVENTION

The armour of falsehood is subtly wrought out of darkness, and hides a man not only from others, but from his own soul.
~ E. M. Forster
A Room With A View

All hell broke loose after Tyler released his secret. By expelling his pent-up rage, his being could no longer handle the intensity that came with releasing the unresolved truth. As if consumed by his pain, my son returned to operating the only way he knew how: by drinking himself into oblivion.

During his soul-cleansing binge after releasing a decade of darkness that had consumed his being, he was inconsolable and physically out of control. Kate frantically texted me that Tyler had just directed pepper spray straight into his own eyes. I believe it was another effort in self-harm. I immediately called her back. I could hear him screaming in the background. Instead of having her automatic compassionate nursing intuition kick in, his girlfriend was getting irritated with him, and I could hear it in her voice. She was heavily exhaling in a huff at the ends of her sentences; I could almost hear her eyes rolling.

It sounds cold but, I could not say I didn't get it. Dealing with a substance abuser is like dealing with an endlessly crying baby or a demented adult; yet to some degree, you know they did this to themselves. In my frantic state, I suggested she take him to the hospital. She told me she was going to put him in the shower, and at that point, we hung up. She called back soon after. He was howling in agony at this point, so she conceded and called EMS.

They quickly arrived with seven police cars. Kate tried to quietly mention that Tyler was self-harming and had mentioned suicidal thoughts, which he had done with her earlier. He happened to overhear her, and he perked up instantly and said, "no sir, I'm fine. I'm not hurting any longer, and I'm not going in the ambulance. I do not want to be taken to the hospital, and I won't go." The horrifying memory and resulting stress from his experience in that Austin hospital will stay with him for a lifetime. After he signed the EMS no-fault liability statement saying he refused transport, they left.

My husband and I, nearly three hours away from him, became desperate. For the first and only time in his career, Alex made the emergency decision to treat Tyler medicinally with Ativan, so there could be some control over the situation. The police, EMS, Kate—they all had tried, but this is what it looks like when someone is in crisis: there is no real solution in that moment, so you do what you have to, and you just do the best you can under those circumstances.

CRISIS INTERVENTION

Kate loaded Tyler into her car and drove to the pharmacy to pick up the controlled medication, the same one routinely used to combat withdrawal in alcohol abusers. Kate got him to take the medication, and eventually, everyone stumbled back to bed, including us. Alex had prescribed nine Ativan pills with instructions to take one every eight hours for three days. This was an intervention to help him remain sedated through the first hurdle of withdrawal and become lucid enough to recognize the need for outside help, which he always had done.

During another sleepless night, I crawled out of bed before dawn and drove to their apartment on the second floor of a historic home in Downtown Wilmington. Once again, I should have allowed natural consequences to occur, but somewhere in my haze, I listened to the voice of un-reason.

I walked into the apartment. My twisted mind of order wouldn't quite compute. The apartment reeked of alcohol, marijuana, and vomit. All I could think of at that moment was why hadn't anyone cleaned up that putrid mess? I found my son in his bed. His clothes from the day before were still on and looked dirty, bunched up, and uncomfortable. He couldn't feel this because he still wasn't feeling much of anything. He was lying on his stomach with his face turned toward the door, and I could see how swollen and red his eyes were from the pepper spray. He was extremely bloated. His lips were inflamed with a bluish-purple hue. His fingers were dirty and puffy, like sausages. He looked like someone pulled from the water after they had drowned.

I checked to make sure he was still breathing. I started crying but swallowed hard because I knew I had to be strong enough to get him the help he needed. People often say parents should never have to bury a child; we should die in the natural order of things, but I can tell you that neither should anyone see their child in the state I witnessed my son in that morning.

Kate was in the family room, curled up in the corner of her couch, wide-eyed with the look of a terrorized animal. I could tell she was desperately trying to pull herself together on my behalf, but on the phone, she hadn't mentioned the shattered vase, the clothes thrown on the floor, the horrid smell, or the empty wine boxes and bottles thrown about. I felt she was traumatized by everything that had happened. We talked for a while. It was the first time, I believe, she understood where I had been coming from when I tried to explain the hardship that lay before her.

A part of me felt like I was dumping my problems at her door, yet she remained adamant about taking care of him and being there for him in spite of my warnings. Maybe the truth is his girlfriend was actually smarter than I was because she recognized her inability to change another human, whereas it took me many years to figure out that simple fact.

Together, Kate and I decided to call a *Crisis Intervention*. The Wikipedia definition of this is a time-limited intervention with a specific psychotherapeutic approach to immediately stabilize those in crisis. What it fails to mention is the person in crisis has to give permission for these qualified individuals to come to them. Tyler was unconscious, so how exactly was that supposed to happen?

After talking to a marginally helpful Crisis Intervention specialist on the phone, we decided it would not work in our situation. I'm not sure how much worse of a crisis situation you can have, but we had to figure something else out. I also knew there was no way I was going to subject him to the traumatizing response of the police and emergency room personnel. I had lost trust in those services for this type of situation a long time ago.

While we were deliberating over our next move, we heard him waking up. He slowly and painfully pulled himself upright in his bed and got up on his feet. We could hear him stumbling in the other room, and we looked at each other with dread. He tried to speak but was incoherent. He staggered into the living room where we were sitting and without acknowledgment, he asked where the alcohol was. He was desperately trying to find it while simultaneously trying to stand. It looked like a comical ballet routine.

Kate and I went into all out-diversion mode. We tried conversing about the cat, which made him stumble to put food in the cat's bowl. If it weren't my son, and his life wasn't in complete shambles, this part would have been just plain funny. It was like watching the movie *Arthur*, a comedy and love story about a drunken New York City billionaire. Unfortunately, nothing about any of this was humorous.

Somehow, with the unrelenting negotiating powers of wine, we simultaneously got him to agree to go to the hospital if I went and got some for him. How ludicrous was this bargaining chip? He took an Ativan, but we knew it would take at least thirty minutes to take effect.

I went into the store and picked up some bread, bananas, a protein bar, some 7-Up and walked over to the wine display. It was still early in the morning. Purchasing wine at 9:00 a.m. seemed completely out of place, so I needed the other food items for it to appear as if I was just picking it all up for the day.

How absurd that I cared or that I was doing the thing I swore I would never do. Yet again I was purchasing the very poison killing my child. I did learn that many years ago, alcohol itself was used medicinally to treat alcohol withdrawal, but somehow that did not make what I went through mentally any easier.

When I got back to the apartment, I walked in with everything in two bags. I continued to distract him for a while. Eventually however, he caught on and asked for his part of the bargain. I reminded him of his agreement. I told him he had to eat a banana before I'd give him the alcohol. Somehow, it was easy to negotiate under these circumstances, and he did what I asked. I got a glass and poured about six ounces in it. I handed it to him, and he drank it like it was shot of hard liquor in a Western movie. He demanded more immediately, so I turned up the negotiating powers, but first I went into the kitchen and poured a good portion of what I thought he wouldn't notice down the drain.

I came back in and put the bottle behind the chair I was sitting in. He started retching and expressing how much pain he was having, so I said it was time to go. He didn't argue. He started crying instead. Kate and I scrambled to get his things together. She promised him she would see him that night as soon as she got to work. This was a huge advantage that worked in our favor. He was so afraid of being taken away to jail or involuntarily committed, so it was monumental that he trusted her in this moment. He demanded that we bring his wine, so I picked up one of the bags and we walked out.

It was a feat just getting him into the car. We started driving and he asked for his chardonnay, which sounds way more elegant that it was at that moment. I handed him the bag I brought, and he looked in to find bread, a protein bar, and 7-Up. "Where's my wine? You didn't bring it?!" he yelled, but at the same time he started vomiting again, so I used the excuse that I accidently grabbed the wrong bag, but it was too late to go back, and we had to get him to the hospital. In his current state, he didn't argue with me.

We arrived at the Emergency Room entrance. I put my face mask on and tried to help him with his, which was futile. He got out of the car but sat on the cold cement directly in front of the door. I helped him up, and we slowly got to the admissions desk. He was having difficulty standing, so I suggested he sit in a chair while I checked him in.

"What is he being seen for?" the person at the front desk asked without really looking up.

I said, "acute alcohol intoxication, and intractable vomiting." I went on to say, "I'm a PA, and all I ask is that my son be treated with dignity in this situation." I was getting quite used to being direct about my expectations.

"Of course, we'll take care of him," she said. "Don't worry."

We both looked over to finalize Tyler's check in, but he wasn't where I left him. She came from behind the desk, and we both frantically started asking the other patients sitting in the ED if they had seen him.

One woman pointed toward the doors and said, "Is that your son you're looking for? I think I saw him go out the front door." I assumed he had bolted from the scene to get more alcohol.

The nurse and I ran out the front doors together and searched in front of the hospital. He wasn't there. We walked toward the parking lot, and my heart was pounding loudly. I turned around toward the nurse and caught a glimpse of him in the corner of my eye directly to the right of the doors. He was down on his knees, curled over on the ground. He was convulsively puking in the grass, only this time, blood was on the ground in front of him.

The nurse yelled for help and snapped at someone to get a wheelchair. We collectively got him in the chair. Blood was coming from his mouth and nose simultaneously. The dark foul angry red was all over his face, hands, and clothes. They wheeled him directly to the back. I wasn't allowed to go with him because of the pandemic. I stood there stunned, not really processing what just happened. I noticed an older man who clearly had some awful illness seated in a wheelchair to my right. I looked at him and could see the pity for me in his eyes. I started crying and shamefully turned around.

I sat in my car and cried for what seemed like hours but was only minutes. Given the condition Tyler was in, I knew no one would be calling me to pick him up any time soon. I decided to drive the forty-five minutes home to the beach. I sat on the couch in the solitude and silence until I passed out from utter exhaustion waiting for the hospital to call with an update.

CHAPTER 15

DETACHED LOVE

> *Just because someone stumbles and loses their path,*
> *doesn't mean they're lost forever.*
> ~ Simon Kinberg
> X-Men: Days of Future Past

It had been hours without any updates, so I called the hospital. They said Tyler was being admitted, just as I had thought. They believed he had a gastric bleed, and by that night, they would be deciding whether they would have to operate. Due to a bed shortage, they kept him in the ED overnight. They made him comfortable with more Ativan. I called Alex and told him to cancel my patients for the following day. He took me out of work for the rest of the week.

The next morning, I assumed Tyler had been admitted by that time, and the newly instituted protocol was a single visitor per patient per hospital stay due to Covid restrictions. I arrived to find that he was still being held in the emergency department. I called the nurses' station to find out what his disposition was. I assumed I was going to have to turn around and drive home. We were in the stage of the pandemic that, due to a healthcare worker shortage, they asked if I was able to sit with my son while still in the ED and watch him instead of a paid *babysitter*. I gladly accepted the job. His girlfriend had also visited him the night before when she took a break from her responsibilities.

We all altered our lives all the time for him.

He stayed there, with me at his bedside, for the rest of the day. He was getting antsy and would be given his *get me through withdrawal without feeling anything* medicines when a nurse would happen to be available, which wasn't very often. The overcrowding due to Covid was hard to witness. It made me grateful for the primary care environment I worked in.

Tyler was finally admitted around seven or eight o'clock that night. I went to his room for just a few minutes, kissed him on his forehead, and told him I would be back in the morning. I would have stayed, had I been allowed, but it was likely better for both of us that I took the chance to go home. I left in a daze and felt drunk on this hard, unforgiving life I had been given.

Tyler was asleep in his hospital bed the next morning, and his phone was ringing off the hook. To avoid the loud ringer waking him up—I was always concerned with his needs and feelings before my own—I picked up his phone and instinctively answered it. It was Sean, his biological father. I hadn't spoken to him in over three years. He was married to a woman who was routinely cruel to my son, manipulative to my ex-husband, and quite hateful toward me,

DETACHED LOVE

so communication with them was not a priority. I had tried to reach out to Tyler's father many times, but he always told me what was happening was Tyler's problem, and they were not going to buy in to it. Sean and his wife were doing the tough love approach. I always felt that he had abandoned his son, and I carried a thousand tons of resentment around because of it. That was all the way up until right then, when I told him over the phone in the hallway of the hospital the truth about what happened to Tyler.

His father said, "no, no, no," and cried, and then, just as I had done, the questions started coming: *when, who, where, why?*

I tried to fill him in to the best of my minimal knowledge. I was worried Tyler would wake up and hear me talking to his dad and telling him something I had no idea if he wanted me to reveal. I felt it was critically important that I tell Sean, like I had told my mom, that it wasn't all Tyler's fault. I wanted them to know he had been hurt so badly and was carrying an amount of shame no one outside of his brain could remotely understand.

It was completely misplaced shame, but that's not something a victim can always understand. But it gave me the right to essentially say, "You were wrong, Sean."

I wasn't trying to hold this over him in the least. I only wanted him to find the compassion for his son he had failed to provide all those years. I wanted him to show up, damn it, like Alex had always done. I wanted him to recognize that he needed to be a father all along. As for my mom, I wanted her to also know that Tyler wasn't the black sheep of the family that he always felt he was. I wanted her to know the brutality of what happened to him, so that I wasn't the only one hurting to know such things. Tyler never woke up during my conversation with his dad, but, as it turns out, he would be hearing from his dad soon enough.

After three days and multiple visits from various specialists, I took Tyler from the hospital and brought him home to the beach. Kate and I decided it would be best for him to be looked after since she would be working nightshift, and I had already been taken off my schedule. I'm not sure if my son appreciated the situation, but he didn't argue, and we got through the next few days of his recovery.

I spent five straight hours on the phone the day after he came home, scheduling all his follow-up doctor's visits. I'm embarrassed to say I did this, because I should have let him do it on his own. I have to say that the mental health system was remarkably difficult to navigate even for me, who works in healthcare. I felt that in his post-hospitalized state, he wasn't necessarily in a position to figure out this difficult landscape; however, it still wasn't my job to do it. I shouldn't have, and I later told him I never would again. This was one more lesson learned along a very distressed road.

Kate picked up Tyler on his third day of recovery. He went home scared of his new pancreatitis diagnosis and resolved to quit drinking. He stayed sober for twenty-nine days.

Upon learning of Tyler's trauma, my husband developed a more compassionate understanding of what my son was up against. He began to comprehend the mental damage that had been done. Once we knew Tyler was drinking again, we stayed with him to help him through withdrawal, yet again. We watched him together, and Alex was able to talk Tyler though a few cravings using visualization. We had a single Ativan from his previous nine-pill prescription, so we gave him the very last one. He calmed down considerably, and my husband left for the three-hour trip home because he had to get back to work the next morning.

I stayed with Tyler. I slept on their hard and unforgiving Salvation Army recliner and Tyler was on a couch donated from the same source. Their kitty, Beethoven, slept on my lap most of the night, but it was nonetheless turbulent. Tyler tossed and turned like a fish. I woke up nearly every fifteen minutes to check on him. In the morning, his girlfriend arrived home after work. I left. He continued drinking.

By the end of the next week, Kate told Tyler he needed to start Intensive Outpatient Therapy if they were going to make things work. I stepped in, telling them both he could stay with me at the beach house until IOP started on Monday to sober up. I hoped he would have that miraculous intervention that parents constantly pray for, and that one miracle person would change his course forever. I picked him up at his place. Everyone knows you can't trust an alcoholic to drive themselves anywhere because, of course, they'll stop to drink before they arrive.

He had his bags packed and ready to go when I got there. This is very atypical for my son, who rarely thinks ahead. I initially asked him to drive because I had been on the road four hours at that point, and I was exhausted. He gave me that look I know too well. I asked him if he had been drinking and he boldly said, "Yes, that's why I can't drive." At least he had that level of awareness, and I appreciated his honesty.

Tyler ran upstairs when we got home and said he was putting his things in his room before helping me put the groceries away. I knew then that he had brought his contraband along with him. I put up the groceries and asked him to walk the dogs. He did so without the first argument. As soon as he stepped out, I went into his room upstairs and found three boxed white wines. I hid them. It took just a short time until he figured out they were gone and yelled at me about being a *grown-ass adult* who can make his own decisions. In more ways than one, he was right.

He didn't speak to me the rest of that evening. I stayed downstairs and watched TV. I knew he was upstairs in his room for a good part of the evening, but eventually I went to bed. I decided that night that I was *done*.

I was done, and I am done.

I have no idea where my epiphany came from, but that night, it set itself in stone, once and for all. It took far too long for me to come to that realization. I have made more mistakes than I can ever count, but I'm happy I finally saw the light I needed to see. I will never stop loving my child. That sweet, caring, giggly, goofy, humorous, giving, and spiritual young man.

I typically would have gone upstairs after our silent night and tried to talk to him—to be the voice of reason. *Oh please. Who was I kidding?* I had no more reasoning than drying cement had. On this day, however, I stayed downstairs and did the things I needed to catch up on. Eventually he came down and casually talked to me about nothing in particular. I responded as if all was well in the world. We watched a movie together that night like we had done a thousand times before.

The next day, when I finally heard him get up, I let him come around and get his breakfast and some coffee. When I knew he was alert, I said, "I recognize that I have become addicted to controlling you and trying to control your outcome. I have become as unhealthy as you are, and I can't do it anymore. We have tried every imaginable thing to help you, but you have to be the one to help you.

"You know who to call when you need to talk to someone, and that doesn't have to be me. You have fifty people I know of you could call right at this minute, and they would come to your rescue, and I know you know that. I can't be that person anymore. I will never, under any circumstances, abandon you, and if you call me, I will be there to help in a healthy and productive way if your goal is sobriety, but I won't do what I've done here anymore. I'm gonna take you home today and let you figure out if you want to stay sober enough to go to IOP tomorrow. It's not up to me. Your consequences have to be yours."

I later added—because, of course, I have to say unnecessary things and I was still processing my anger—that I felt he had given his previous girlfriend the very best of himself when he was sober, yet she treated him terribly, and now he was with a lovely young woman who adored him and wanted to take care of him, and he was giving her the very worst of himself. I said very directly, "She met you and fell in love with you when you were sober. She fell in love with your authentic self." He didn't respond, just looked down.

We decided to stop for some food on the way home. It all seems too normal to say that, but our relationship enabled some normalcy. We were okay with each other saying what needed to be said. Besides, he was sober, and we were both hungry. We went for some Mexican food. We kept our conversation light initially, but after a while I noticed how badly his hands were shaking. I put his hands in mine from across the table and tried to hold them still, if only for a moment. My heart was weeping, but he didn't see it.

At that moment, I said, "I can't handle it anymore, wondering if it's the last time I'm going to see you."

He simply replied, "I can't handle having this disease anymore."

I just nodded and said I understood. I dropped him off and drove the three agonizing hours home in silent tears.

CHAPTER 16

THE COST OF ADDICTION

Loving an addicted child is like grieving his death and fighting for his life at the same time. All the while hated, helpless, and alone.

~ Anonymous

In total, my husband and I paid for the services of six attorneys, six hospital stays, nine rehabilitation facilities, three post high school education attempts, more than ten detoxes, seven intensive outpatient programs, and at least eight counselors or psychologists. We purchased multiple vehicles, got those vehicles out of the towing yard or paid for major vehicle repairs, paid for rent, electric, phone and cable bills, bank overdraft fees, medical bills, plane tickets, hotel rooms, rental cars, and many, many meals.

At least these are the things I remember paying for. The math adds up very high very quickly. I do not regret spending any of it. I would probably do it again, knowing what I knew then, which was, quite frankly, nothing. It was part of my addiction to the control. I was trying to purchase his survival. If we could purchase that, there would be no loss in the world.

I recognize it was a privilege to be able to financially manage these situations, but that misses the point completely. I never gave him the opportunity to handle any of it independently. It took too long to figure out I was doing it all wrong. I am very intentional now about giving my son any bills that happen into our mailbox and letting him know what I won't do any longer. In other words, I can express my boundaries.

The cost to me and my husband professionally, personally, and even physically was certainly something we couldn't have prepared for. I ultimately became an anxious, frenzied mess of a person. I didn't sleep; I didn't show up for work. Not showing up to see the patients who were scheduled with me was heartbreaking. I know they took time off of work or manipulated their schedules to come in and take care of their own health. I have some very forgiving patients, but a few who just couldn't see past it, and that's just how it had to be.

My stress manifested itself into physical symptoms. My thyroid broke as a result. I ended up with hyperthyroidism and thyroid eye disease. Later I got something known only to the medical books apparently, called *burning mouth syndrome*. It's a phenomenon of being overly stressed. The cost also affected my back and my neck, setting up chronic pain in those areas. I ended up with crushing headaches and ulcers in my stomach and small intestines. In part, I could recognize the costs from having witnessed them in my patients with loved ones who carried this affliction. They regularly had uncontrolled high blood pressure, heart disease, and I'm pretty sure there has to be something known as *broken heart syndrome*, because I witnessed it all the time. Stress *can* kill you, and my patients and I were letting ourselves die a little more every day.

The cost to your marriage, your friendships or other relationships, your job, and your mental health are all greatly overlooked. So much gets lost along the path. You desperately try to hold on to these familiar sources of comfort while simultaneously pushing them away. It's a destructive tug of war, and people around you become exhausted in the process. You can barely hold up—so how can you expect anyone else to manage the constant defeat?

I fortunately had found a man who could withstand punch after punch. We came to realize the damage done to us as a couple and did everything we could to uplift our relationship in spite of the tornado all around us. Most importantly, we communicated. We had to have difficult but brutally honest conversations. It is hard work, but you can't let go of the very people trying to save you while you're trying to save someone else. It's such a tangled web.

If you can step out of your situation and look at it from a distant vantage point, hopefully you'll be able to recognize all you are doing to yourself and those around you before you lose everything, or at least as much as your addicted loved one has lost. There's not a scientific method for your recovery. There's not a perfect plan, but there are resources, and they can make a world of difference. You have to force yourself to tap in to them because no one will do it for you. As each new day comes to pass, you will see the changes you are searching for. Your changes can have the power to manifest your loved one's change.

CHAPTER 17

RECOVERY

Hope is definitely not the same thing as optimism. It is not the conviction that something will turn out well, but the certainty that something makes sense, regardless of how it turns out.

~ Vaclav Havel

I may be pulling back the curtain here, but I have dedicated an entire chapter to finding the right recovery placement because it is, quite frankly, daunting and overwhelming. It can feel like learning the customs of a foreign country for the first time.

I am an advocate for substance use disorder rehabilitation because, in cases like my son's, the multiple treatment facilities were a part of saving his life and educating him about the disease he will have for the rest of his life. It helped his dad and me learn a tremendous amount of integral information as well. This does not mean substance abuse treatment facilities are the only solution. In some cases, they ultimately prove to be bad choices or bad facilities. That is precisely why I wanted to help sort through the maze of information when it comes to making such an important choice for a loved one or yourself.

My son attended rehab nine times, and it took me as many times to finally comprehend the staggering complexity of choosing the right place for him. Tyler attended a wilderness program, stuck it out at a state-funded facility, thrived at a private facility, walked out against medical advice at another location, and wandered unknowingly into unimaginable places within the varying systems. We were as blind as he was when figuring these places out. He had no concept of where to begin. We were the adults having to make the choices in the bleakest of moments.

Under duress describes how you can feel when trying to make such a critical decision for your loved one. It's not likely that you'll have the luxury to step back and give yourself plenty of time to investigate your choices. It is also not like searching on Airbnb for a lovely new place to rent because nobody is *planning* their next rehab stay. The reality is, your loved one is in need *right now*, and they momentarily decide they are willing to give hospitalization a try. Now what?

These are the factors to consider when choosing a rehab facility for your loved one. Hold on tight because the list—in no particular order—is large; however, it is not exhaustive:

1. Price
   - Insurance coverage
   - Out-of-pocket expenses
   - State funded, no insurance necessary, no out-of-pocket expenses
   - Private facility

2. Treatment type
   - Dual diagnosis: SUD combined with underlying mental health or trauma
   - Substance-only treatment
   - Detox
   - DOC (drug of choice)-focused facility (e.g. alcohol, fentanyl, opioids)

3. Treatment modalities
   - Cognitive Behavioral Therapy (CBT)
   - Dialectical Behavior Therapy (DBT)
   - Mindfulness-based Cognitive Therapy
   - Eye Movement Desensitization and Reprocessing (EMDR)
   - Biofeedback
   - Trauma focused
   - Medication assisted

4. Counseling
   - Individual counseling availability: daily, weekly, or semi-weekly
   - Group counseling

5. Licensing, accreditation, and affiliations
   - JCAHO: Joint Commission on Accreditation of Healthcare Organizations
   - CARF: Commission on Accreditation of Rehabilitation Facilities
   - ASAM: American Society of Addiction Medicine
   - SAMHSA: Substance Abuse and Mental Health Services Administration

6. Location
   - Consider visitation
   - Consider family meetings, therapy offered within facility
   - Season/temperature for outdoor activities
   - Proximity to home, to avoid the probability of being able to walk out

7. Approach
   - 12-Step Facilitation: AA and NA
   - SMART Recovery: Self-Management and Recovery Training
   - Religious-based versus secular approach
   - Co-ed versus male/female/other focused

8. Transitional Resources offered
   - Housing: sober living
   - Job searches and placement assistance
   - Establish counseling services, trauma therapy
   - Primary healthcare services
   - Legal services as needed
   - Money management assistance

9. Other factors
   - Outcome data: measurable outcomes related to the treatment approach of the facility
   - LGBTQIA friendly
   - Cleanliness of facility
   - Dietary program
   - Exercise and meditation availability

- Treatment of military PTSD
- Recommendation from local medical providers

As far as reviews are concerned, read them with a grain of salt, and remember those writing them are sometimes the addicted individual not ready to truly recover. However, sometimes negative reviews are simply due to a rehab center being poorly run.

Every rehabilitation facility will have an admission coordinator under varying titles, and they are exceptionally well-trained sales people. They have a knack of telling you want you want to hear in a moment of desperation. It is best to be equipped with information so you can make clear, researched decisions free of less-than-credible influences.

You also need to understand from the start that if your loved one is over the age of eighteen, they are considered an adult and will need to sign a release of information for you to know anything about their time in residence. The facility will not be able to tell you if the patient has left against medical advice, even if you are paying for their treatment. It is pretty controversial because on one hand, there is HIPPA compliance for the facility, and the other, there is the safety of the individual who can leave without your knowledge.

Here's where natural consequences and death-defying actions cross paths, so I personally don't agree with not notifying the family of a patient's unanticipated departure. If you know they are there because you dropped them off yourself, you should have the right at least to know whether they have left. Some treatment centers are forthcoming with this information, and not all fall into the same facility-imposed requirements.

Once you arrive with your loved one at the facility, they will need to fulfill an intake procedure. *I do not encourage you to be a part of this process.* It is difficult to hear the reality of your loved one's past, and in most cases, it all comes pouring out at this interview. You can handle the payment side of things while your loved one completes their intake process. Of course, this is only from the perspective of a family member being part of the admissions process. If you are admitting yourself on your own, it may appear somewhat different.

Then you just leave your loved one behind and drive away. If your loved one was in the hospital you would, under most circumstances, be staying with them, bedside, until they recovered. However, here they stay and, in many cases, begin the gut-wrenching and even dangerous process of detoxing, typically up to seven days. In most cases, they will have their phone taken away, and you will not be able to communicate with them for whatever amount of time is determined by the facility, and then, only on a restrictive basis.

It turns out to be a healing process for all parties involved. They are under the influence of detoxifying medications and asleep a good portion of that first week, and you get to actually sleep soundly without the worry of your loved one out in the world, under the influence or lost. It helps to re-center your universe, without all the chaos and confusion, if only for a short while.

After your loved one is settled in a placement, you may hear status updates from them or their counselor, assuming your loved one has given permission for you to be informed. A decent facility will have communicated with the family fairly early on, however, with staffing shortages and overwhelming admissions, it can be a challenge. My advice is to be patient. As long as you know they are still there and safe, let the facility do their job, and let go of the control that was likely part of the picture all along.

Once your loved one has detoxed and is starting to come around, they'll move into the main house or facility where the work they came for is supposed to happen. They eat, sleep, exercise and participate in group therapy daily from then on, with consistent patients and staff. They become extraordinarily close with other patients because these are the most intimate and vulnerable experiences they will have. The intention is to lay bare their soul, their secrets, their indiscretions, their hopes and dreams for a better life for themselves. Their community becomes these people. They build valuable bonds that can help them well beyond their time at the treatment center if they are true to their fight for sobriety.

These centers can house anywhere from fewer than ten people to several hundred. Tyler participated in both environments. The time the patients spend together is anywhere from one month to one year, or even longer. Although some places are spa-like and cater to wealthy individuals with substance use disorder, they are not all intended to be as such. These are essentially rehabilitation hospitals. If you broke your hip in a car accident, after surgery, you would be taken to a rehab facility to heal first, then learn to walk again. This is not a lot different, and the time after hospitalization isn't exactly a cake walk either—just ask anyone with mending hip replacements. Substance use disorder doesn't just magically disappear after rehab, and truly, the effort only just begins in the *real world* at that point.

Here is where the options of IOP—intensive outpatient therapy— individual counseling, and sober living present themselves. Make no mistake, these factors are just as critical in the decision making as the facility you started with.

Intensive outpatient gives the individual the option of continuing the group and counseling services without living in the facility. This enables the person to work and live back in their homes with their family while still receiving intensive treatment.

Your loved one can also choose to live in a sober living home; sometimes this *choice* is mandated by the court system. Here your loved one will live with other individuals with substance use disorder. You or your loved one typically pay for their room, so the divided rent does support a reduced cost of living; however, there are expectations of participation. Residents are typically expected to take part in weekly drug testing, group meetings, AA or NA, and shared clean-up and cooking.

If the house is authentic, there are no exceptions to the designated rules laid out upon entry. Some sober living homes have poor reputations of continued substance use and no followed rules. These are not where you want your loved one if they are truly desiring a life free of substance abuse. Typically, the only acceptable substances allowed are caffeine and cigarettes. The average sober living homes will not allow suboxone or methadone treatments. Their prohibition of drugs might go so far as including attention deficit stimulant medications.

Individual counseling is also a personal option after leaving a treatment facility. It can certainly aid in the prolonged success of SUD remission and provide lifelong resources for continued abstinence.

Tyler brought up something of great value while attending different treatment facilities. The only places he had any measurable success was at the facilities where he felt respected. He often noticed that, independent of the patients' age, status, or educational level, they were regularly "talked down to," in his words, at certain treatment centers. He made the comment that he already felt less than human just by being there. Then to be "treated like a child" was too much, and he would often bow out at that point.

On the other hand, he experienced several occasions when the opposite occurred. One facility in Arizona was especially respectful to the patients and treated them from an educated perspective. It is no secret that individuals with SUD complete the spectrum of education and intelligence. Being treated and spoken to with mutual respect works in nearly every situation, so why wouldn't it work in a substance treatment facility? Turns out, it does.

After rehab, intensive outpatient treatment, and sober living comes life back in the fast lane. The goal is to continue to live without the aid of their drug-of-choice, which for many had been their most well-worn coping mechanism. Our job is to be kind, be respectful, and be helpful when our loved ones need our assistance. If they have come to understand that nothing in this life is achieved alone, our help is exactly what they will need and want.

CHAPTER 18

TAKE CARE

> *I have come to believe that caring for myself is not self-indulgence, it is self-preservation.*
> ~ Audre Lorde
> A Burst of Light and Other Essays

There is a reason you are told to put *your* mask on before helping a loved one when a plane is in duress. If you shrivel up and become useless, so will everything around you. You have to make a profound and conscious decision to put in the work on *you*, so you can put in the tireless work that will be required of you for *them*. How in the hell can you even get out of the bed in order to do what I'm saying right now? Throw the covers back and put one foot at a time on the floor and push yourself up. Every action will be a challenge initially, but it will get easier.

Write, scream, breathe, ask for help; do whatever it takes. You deserve to make it. <u>You deserve yet another day</u>, another try, another sunset, just as much as that person with this sickening disease does. So, step one is *get up*.

Stop Ruminating

When I say <u>*ruminating,*</u> I mean <u>*cyclic thinking*</u>—when you simply can't stop the recurring thought pattern that keeps you frozen and unable to develop solutions or heal yourself. For the longest time, I checked off the self-care list of items as if they were chores. I told myself I was doing what I was supposed to be doing, but to be honest, I wasn't. The entire time, I was ruminating about him.

I wasn't on a walk while listening to music, I was walking with music in my ears and a monologue in my head that sounded like: *Why hasn't he texted me back yet? Maybe I should text him again, or actually I'll just call him. If he doesn't answer but it rings several times, then I know his phone is on at least. If I text him and the text message comes up as delivered than his phone is still on which means he likely was sober enough to plug it in and recharge the battery.* <u>But if the word</u> *Delivered* didn't appear under the message, the <u>anxiety would kick</u> in. I would wait an indeterminate amount of time, usually until I just couldn't take the worry anymore, and I would then try to call.

If it went right to voicemail, then assumptions kicked in all at once: *His phone is dead. He never plugged it in because he was blacked out. Maybe he's dead. Maybe he's in jail. Maybe he's on the streets and has nowhere to charge his phone. Is he hungry, cold, alone?* Maybe I had become completely deranged and let these thoughts creep in unabated. I couldn't stop catastrophizing. I wasn't taking care of myself or my own mental health. I was completely defeated. The ruminating thoughts of his life had taken over my life.

The more I pretended to take care of myself, the more of a lie it became. I needed to see the ridiculous things I was doing before actual self-care could take place. I would start with the prayers begging God to have Tyler call me, as if God does this type of ludicrous request on the spot. Surprisingly, nearly every single time I asked, Tyler called within a short time, and I took a breath and went on with my day, worrying at my baseline with the thought-circus playing in the back of my head—the internal dialogue perpetuated by chronic fear. I worried whether he was functional, blacked out, with horrible people, on the street, in his car, without his phone, clean, hungry, or alive. I worried if his teeth were still in his head or if he had gotten into a fight and gotten them knocked out again. I worried he would get run over or kill someone else with his car.

I ruminated over every question and every step in my head a thousand times. Every minute step over the many eggshells we attempted to avoid all the time, and every question we asked a thousand times in a loop in our head.

Should I say what I want to say?
Should I call him right now or later?
Should I answer the phone when he calls?
Should I go look for him?
Should I bail him out of jail?
Should I help him financially?
Should I ask if he's using?
Should I call the police?
Should I make excuses for him?

Should I call his friends?
Should I tell him I know he's lying?
Should I believe him when I think he's actually telling the truth?

Along with a million other questions, these can swim around in your brain, causing unbearable anxiety, dread, and anger. They can keep you riding a dangerous rollercoaster. I rode an actual rollercoaster called The Beast when I was a teenager. Little did I know it would become the presage of my life.

I stopped being aware of anything else in my life but him. My husband felt my absence, my patients likely felt my distance, and my family and friends felt the space I placed between us. I was so involved in worrying that I wasn't even aware of life going on around me most of the time. I completely stopped taking care of myself. I was living solely through him.

Get Help

In order to get it together at the most basic level, I first recognized what I was doing. *Hi, I'm Lisa and I'm a controlaholic.* Once that came into crystal clear focus, the rest unfolded quite easily. I got help. I started seeing a therapist, and I started taking an anti-depressant during that time. This is something I swore I would never do because I never thought I'd need to, plain and simple. I assumed I could just handle it. I was so wrong. The medication didn't take away the pain; it just mitigated the deep despair and gave me some room to think critically. It gave me the ability to focus and to stop the cyclic, downward-spiral thinking that kept me glued to my thoughts born out of fear. It may not be the reckoning for everyone, but it sure got me to a better place than I had been in for way too long.

I combined my counseling and antidepressant with exercise and writing. This became my formula for revival. My own rebirth needed to happen because I was being swallowed whole by the disease of addiction. I was fading into an oblivion no one would be able to rescue me from. After many years, I went through a phase, similar to the dry drunk, when I made a conscious decision to live my life to the fullest in between crises. I learned to compartmentalize my time. When my son was sober, or at least safe, I put my full effort into my husband, my work, my friends, my hobbies, and myself. I experienced those events and relationships as if the world were in perfect order. I really did remain present. When Tyler wasn't sober, however, all my energy and focus went solely to him. This was effective for a short while, but I was living a complete lie, and it was never going to be sustainable, nor was it healthy or helpful to anyone. I felt I was always waiting for the other shoe to drop.

Go to Group Therapy

I found understanding—and most importantly at that time, a lack of judgment—from group therapies such as AA, SMART Recovery, and Thrive Family Support. They are all tremendously helpful but work very differently for different people. I am such an internal thinker that, after a while, it became difficult to get the words I needed to speak in the group meetings and left me more frustrated at times. I came to realize that whatever outlet works for you is the one to use throughout this process. People will say you *have* to attend the meetings, but if the meetings aren't really working for you, try something else for a while, then come back and try again later, or try a completely different style of meeting.

As much of an independent as I am, I have to admit the value of groups. They are a safety net when it feels like the whole universe just doesn't understand. There is nothing you can say to the people in these meetings that they won't be able to relate to. I remember meeting people of a higher socio-economic level who believed they were above these meetings for some reason. I'm here to tell you there isn't a more stripped-down human experience than this pain, and no number of possessions can separate anyone from it.

I walked into my first-ever Al-Anon meeting in Austin. The facility was some random building, like the kind where we used to have family reunions at the park. It was dark with wood paneling. One side was evidently for AA because I accidently went in that direction, and apparently, I looked very out of place because someone quickly said, "Are you looking for the Al-Anon group? They're right over there."

I walked across the main gathering room and into the abyss. People were filing in with smiles and hugs, and all I could do was hold my breath and bite my tongue to keep myself from crying and running out of there. I sat down in the first chair I could slip into without being noticed.

A mother and her son were getting settled next to me, and I could overhear them talking about his impending court case and jail time. He must have realized I was within earshot of their conversation because he looked up at me with a huge smile on his face and tried to explain that he was facing a seven-year prison sentence for a drug-fueled offense. He was grateful, almost gleeful, to be telling me his story and how lucky he was to have the chance to redeem himself.

His mother was less than full of joy but not as sad as I would have expected her to be. Maybe it was simply because of her son's sobriety and healing, even though he was facing jail time. We've all been there: In some ways, hoping they'll be in jail because at least they're not dead. We know where they are, and we know they have to be sober. What a horrible thing to have to hope for.

The room began to quiet down, and I could feel that enormous lump in my throat just aching to be released by tears. One person started the session and asked if there were any newcomers. I reluctantly raised my hand, but books and pamphlets were placed in it with several words of warm welcome. The standard start to the meeting, the ten-step Al-Anon prayer began, and I listened intently but with a mixture of sadness, anger, and fear.

After the topic was determined and a few passages were read, an attractive, middle-aged man spoke up. He just wasn't the kind of guy I expected to see at a meeting, even though I have no idea what I was expecting. I was calmed by his presence. He told the story of his twin daughters and their long-term addiction. He then went on to talk about their subsequent, multiple hospital visits. One night he was called by EMS telling him his daughter was in the emergency department after a drug- and alcohol-related incident. She was okay, but she was, nonetheless, there. He rushed to the hospital. At 2:00 a.m., in the hospital waiting room for the umpteenth time, a thought occurred to him: *I spend ninety-nine percent of my time thinking and worrying about my daughter, and she spends all of maybe one percent of her time worried or thinking about me.*

Having realized that, he got up and just left the hospital. He knew he'd be called with an update, so he went back to bed.

That hit me across the face hard enough to leave figurative welts. I was able to swallow the lump in my throat, and I thought: *Oh my God! When is the last time my son even thought about me, about how I was, if I was safe, sad, or healthy?*

I went up to the father of twins after the meeting and said simply, "Thank you. Your words were exactly what I needed to hear." I attended several more times while I was staying in Austin, and I learned a lot. I felt it had real potential to help.

When I went back to North Carolina, I tried Al-Anon close to my home. In my rural community there would be a single meeting per week, per town. In large cities, you can find a meeting nearly every hour of the day, seven days a week.

The difference between the experience in Austin and my hometown was night and day. While there were approximately fifty people in the Al-Anon meeting in Austin, there were maybe seven people at my local meeting. Some had lost their addicted love one years before. One woman routinely fell asleep at the meetings as if no one would be able to notice. After several weeks, I tried to go to a different meeting in a different town, and I was the only one in attendance. I kind of gave up, and at the same time, my son went into remission. I actually thought: *Hallelujah, my son is all better! I don't ever have to go to another Al-Anon meeting.* Of course, that's just not how it works.

I began my relationship with Al-Anon very pissed off. Why did I have to go if he had the problem? I was busy. (I'd pretend.) I have other plans. (I didn't.) It was just not fair. (What is?)

The pandemic had its silver linings, one of them being Zoom meetings, which I could attend in the comfort of my home whenever I wanted. It got tough sometimes, listening to either the optimist who always had a smile on their face and clichéd their way through everything, or the eternal pessimist who never looked at anything through any other angle. I felt like I'd been on the hamster wheel and that the comments made were on repeat. I felt like my story was different because of the trauma. I believed I couldn't exactly relate to those whose kids were using to use or using because their home life was difficult. These thoughts were borne out of resentment at the time. The truth was our stories weren't any different. We were all down in the same muck together.

In the big scheme of recovery, these groups definitely have their practical value. They are worth your time and effort. Sometimes the lessons gained from them can be priceless. It is beyond valuable just to have a place to speak up and express how you are feeling instead of trying to hold it in all the time. Groups helped get me through some really tough days, and I met some incredible people by participating in this form of help. My hope is that you, too, can acquire what you need within a group of your choice.

Discover Distractions

Whatever self-care looks like to you—painting, jogging, swimming, meditating—I sincerely encourage you to just do it. These are the very things that get pushed aside when we're in the fear zone. We don't believe we deserve these things because *how in God's name can I paint when I know my son is on the street and hungry?*

How? You force yourself, and when you start, you recognize that it becomes an outlet that makes the chronic cycle of worry slow down and gives your brain a much-needed rest. Even going on a short walk or calling a friend can have surprisingly healing powers. Would all the worrying in the world change the outcome? Or would the distraction actually feed your soul in a way that helps you carry on?

It sounds impossible, and some days it just will be, but on the days when you can, find a way. There were times when my son was in active addiction, in crisis mode, and when I would sit down to write, it simply helped to divert my chronic suffering and the catastrophizing that I constantly found myself doing. As ironic as it is, I was forced to think about something else.

Exercise, even for the average citizen without a loved one with addiction issues, is difficult to accomplish, but it's as necessary as oxygen. It has multiple benefits besides distraction, which include mood improvement, sleep enhancement, and increased energy at a time when energy feels liked it's being sucked out of you with a Dyson vacuum.

I pushed myself through exercise initially, but now it's my gift to myself that keeps giving. If exercise wasn't in the cards before you started experiencing this whirlwind, it's not like you're going to enjoy it now, so all I can say is get out in the fresh air and just walk. It's meditative without having to meditate, and it expends much needed mental energy so you can stop the tickertape for a while.

Oh yeah—need I mention journaling? Write down anything you can—your hurts, frustrations, or your accomplishments and gratitudes daily. Just getting the thoughts to come out of your swirling head feels like relief, even if it's just enough to be able to fall asleep more easily.

Get Sleep

Speaking of sleep: It is another form of self-care that is absolutely critical in terms of your recovery. It revitalizes the brain and helps your anxiety level stay low. Patient after patient returns to my office to report how much their anxiety improved after they got help with their sleep disorder. The studies confirm this, but there's nothing quite like the empirical accounts to confirm what you already know.

Let's be honest, I know it's not easy to sleep soundly when your loved one has a substance use disorder, but it's a critical necessity for you. This is not about them. *Sleep hygiene*, a medical term, means to create a daily routine and environment that promotes sound, consistent sleep.

Here's a simple guide:
- Avoid screens (TV, computers, phones, and iPads) an hour prior to bedtime
- Avoid large meals, alcohol, and caffeine several hours before going to bed
- Be consistent with bedtime and waketime, including on the weekends
- Exercise during the day to expend energy

I'm not assuming that this can work consistently for you, but get the most from your sleep when you can. Sleep is one of the most powerful medicines we can give ourselves.

Be Realistic and Accepting

On any given day, I'll report a different level of resolve. I wish I could say I soldiered on without faltering in any way, but that's just not the case. Depending on my own amount of sleep, work, and activity, my ability to stick to a plan varied.

One acronym counselors share with patients who live with substance use disorder is HALT, which stands for *Hungry*, *Angry*, *Lonely*, or *Tired*. Check in with yourself when making decisions, and don't make them if one of those feelings is in question. We all know we don't function well when we're hungry or tired, for example. There's also MEPS—an acronym used for asking yourself how you're feeling *Mentally*, *Emotionally*, *Physically*, and *Spiritually* on a regular basis.

These concepts aren't exclusive to the addicted loved ones, they're for us all to apply as part of our own recovery. I know I'm not telling you anything you don't already know to some degree, but you may just need a reminder or push in the right direction. I would strongly encourage you to go as far as to record your daily MEPS in a journal.

Or how about writing a gratitude journal? There were days that I couldn't even feel the joy of not being six feet under. Those were the very days I needed to remind myself of what I had to be thankful for. There *are* other things happening in our lives. There *are* other people in our lives who deserve our attention. I don't mean just our presence, but our actual attention. Most importantly, one of those people is you.

Our recovery is just as critical as theirs. Our survival is just as important as theirs. Our life is just as meaningful as theirs. It's easy to forget these truths when you're lost in the maze of addicted delusions, but <u>you'll never be able to help your loved one until you help yourself.</u> If you simply can't do any of these things, then just read. Educate yourself so that you can arm yourself with knowledge and understanding. When you are strong enough, things will begin to change. If not for them, then for you.

CHAPTER 19

HEALING THROUGH

As soon as that healing takes place, then we have to go out and heal somebody . . . so somebody else gets it and passes it on.
~ Maya Angelou, interviewed in
Maya Angleou's I Know Why the Caged Bird Sings: A Casebook

I looked across the exam room and observed another distraught mother—weary eyes underscored by dark drawn circles from lack of sleep and chronic worry—asking for help due to her daughter's addiction as I reflected on the reality of the epidemic. Not the viral pandemic that so many had been frustrated by in 2020 to 2023, but the substance abuse epidemic and lack of readily available information to those who need it most. We have truly come so far in the understanding of mental health, and substance use disorder, but there is still so much to learn.

Political change is happening and has been since Patrick Kennedy's mental health bill initiative—the Mental Health Parity and Addiction Equity Act, passed in 2008—that changed our understanding and treatment of these conditions. President Barack Obama later designed an initiative to fully provide health coverage for those suffering with mental health or substance use disorders equivalent to those with cardiovascular disease or diabetes. Yet, when I talk to the families of my patients, they remain completely lost when it comes to simple, readily available resources they so desperately need. I write out my long list for them of where they can access the many resources at their disposal. I've shared this list below. As I've said, it took ten years to accumulate the information I've provided. My hope is that it can impact your circumstances sooner than it did mine.

This is a fairly exhaustive list with brief descriptions. My family and I tried many of them, but I don't want to provide an opinion about their efficacy because everything has the potential to work under different circumstances. I want you to know what's available and what your loved one may have access to. I do not want individuals to have to scramble for years trying to figure out the road map to recovery. There are many routes, and having knowledge is having power.

FOR THEM:

Treatment Facilities

Intensive Outpatient Therapy (IOP): Patients with substance use disorder go to a designated location for up to three hours a day, at least three days per week, for group and individual therapy and counseling.

Inpatient detox center: These are medically supervised centers only for addicted individuals who are or have the possibility of experiencing the serious and potentially deadly effects of substance withdrawal. Medications such as benzodiazepines (Xanax, Ativan, Valium), anti-seizure medications, and anti-nausea meds are administered for up to seven days in certain patients. A medical professional is always available and is responsible for monitoring your loved one's vitals and health during their stay.

Inpatient residential rehabilitation: Typically overseen by a medical doctor, this is a location that houses individuals with substance use disorder, usually for a minimum of thirty days. I actually knew a patient who was sure all inpatient rehabs were just like jail, and you were made to stay there against your will. This is definitely not the case at all, and the truth is, your loved one can walk away at their discretion. That is important to know.

In reality, the patients sleep, eat, and attend sessions all day, every day, with each other. They attend group therapy and individual counseling. They can also work out or just rest. There are many different types of inpatient rehab. Straight addiction treatment was at one time the most common, but dual diagnosis treatment centers have become considerably more popular. *Dual diagnosis* means both the addiction and the underlying mental health or trauma-related symptoms are being treated. Some treatment centers are free, and the patients are required to work at a job while there for up to two years. Some centers revolve around equine therapy or farming. Some are wilderness or outdoor treatment centers, where your loved one spends time in the woods and learns to rely on themself. Sometimes trauma counseling, EMDR, CBT-type therapies, among others, are provided.

It takes a village to find the right place for your loved one, so don't leave it solely up to them. If they're ready to make the commitment—which is a huge deal and has the potential to be a short-lived desire of theirs—it's typically not while they are in the most conscious state, so they will need your help. I encourage doing research on inpatient rehabilitation based on location, cost, insurance coverage, and approach or methods of treatment. It takes time and a lot of questioning over the phone, but it comes down to the commitment of the individual and their true desire for sobriety.

Sober living home: These settings are typically associated with the inpatient residential facility, meaning the facilities are usually well acquainted with the local sober homes. They can be donation based or self-pay or private. Some of these homes charge a weekly or monthly rent for a bedroom in an established sober home with a set number of other residents sharing the common goal of staying sober. In most cases, there is no time limit on a resident's stay, and they can choose to leave at their will.

This can truly be transformative. Having the freedom in recovery while being surrounded by people going through the same challenges can make all the difference. My son stayed in a sober home with individuals who were married or had children—they stayed in sober living while family members remained living at home.

The amount of connection, accountability, and support in a sober home can change an outcome. Residents are typically required to pass breathalyzer tests and drug screenings on a consistent basis. In most cases, they would be asked to leave or removed if they failed a test. Residents are typically required to attend recovery meetings as well. Some homes are very well kept, have high rents, and dedicated residents, but where there is a yin, there is always a yang, so it's wise to do some research before signing any type of residential contract.

Halfway house or *residential re-entry centers:* These are very similar to sober living homes, but stays are typically court mandated or state sponsored after incarceration. There may be a limit on the amount of time a resident is allowed to stay. The resident has to pay rent and pass drug tests, but they may also be under the control of the legal system by way of a parole officer or other means.

Counseling/Life Coaching

Psychiatrists: These practitioners manage psychiatric medications. They are not who you are looking for if you desire counseling, but they will determine the best medication or combination of medications to meet the needs of a person with substance use disorder or combined mental health disorders.

Psychologists: These focus on investigative work or studies. They perform assessments for ADHD, autism, learning disabilities, and IQ, but they're not ideal for discussing issues. These individuals can also be helpful for patients with a suspected Traumatic Brain Injury or TBI. Specifically, a *neuropsychologist* can be of help in this area. It's best to call a practice to find out if they meet your loved one's counseling needs.

Counselors: They come in many shapes and sizes. One of the better resources is www.psychologytoday.com. Once you've pulled up the website, click the Find a Therapist link. You can filter by your issues, your insurance, your location, practitioner's gender, and so many other things, so it narrows results to exactly what you are looking for in your precise area of the country. In addition, there are now multiple apps available to connect with a counselor for your specific concerns by simply using your phone.

Primary Care Provider (PCP): Get one immediately. They are essential for monitoring your loved one's overall physical health, but they are also someone to be accountable to. Showing up for appointments can become an important part of recovery. PCPs check your vitals and labs regularly. A substance abuser can have physiological changes without having overt symptoms, and regular appointments can serve as lifesaving interventions.

Sober companion: This is a potentially expensive option for someone to be present as a type of life coach, motivator, distractor, and friend in the exhaustive process of recovery. They can live with your loved one or be regularly available. They help establish healthy routines and give encouragement through early sobriety. During a global pandemic, for instance, they may just be the difference between success and continued use.

Medications

Before I list medications, please know there is something called a PHQ-9. This is an easily downloadable test to assess for depression and the need for possible medication. The moral of the story is it's a personal choice to try medication. I've seen significant changes in some people I've started on antidepressants, and others, not much change at all. There are typically complicating features in those individuals, such as personality disorders or bipolar disorder. Effexor (venlafaxine), for example, has an additional off-label indication to treat ADD and evidence to support its benefit in treating substance use disorder. It is critical to talk with a healthcare provider about your need for medication and the available choices.

One study conducted in 1999 compared the effects of three months of exercise to three months of medication and showed similar outcomes in reduction of symptoms of depression, among other findings (Duke University 1999). There are many available treatment options to consider if deciding to go down this path.

Medication Assisted Treatment (MAT): This simply means using medication to assist the goal of sobriety. It has a bit of controversy associated with it because the goal is typically to be substance free, but your loved one has to do what works best for them, and that may be with Campral, for example. This would be in combination with all the other resources available.

Antidepressants: These are daily medications taken to relieve the symptoms of depression or anxiety or both in conditions such as major depressive disorder and generalized anxiety disorder. They also help treat obsessive compulsive disorder, panic disorder, and post-traumatic stress disorder or PTSD. Some of these medications, such as Cymbalta, also have an indication to treat pain. The list of these medications is very long, so it is best to discuss options with a healthcare provider. There are also companies like Genomind and GeneSight that do genetic testing specifically for mental health disorders to analyze the best treatment options for a patient based on their specific DNA. I did this for my son and appreciated what we learned from the testing.

Mood stabilizers: These are used for bipolar disorder, schizophrenia, and treatment resistant depression. Some have off-label indications for alcohol dependence. These are more involved diagnoses that require a mental health specialist.

Opioid antagonist: In pill or injectable forms, Naltrexone and Vivitrol can be used to reduce cravings of opioids or alcohol. They also reduce the euphoric feelings associated with these substances. They can take several weeks before they kick in and reduce cravings. They can only be used after a patient has been opioid free for seven to ten days.

Topiramate (Topamax): Topiramate decreases withdrawal severity and lessens motivation to drink. These are known as *off-label indications*. This means they have not been formally studied in these areas and are not FDA approved but have shown efficacy in post-marketing analysis.

Acamprosate (Campral): This medication is specifically for alcoholism. It works on the brain's neurotransmitters, but its mechanism of action is not completely understood. It can reduce the desire to drink. This is most effective in people who are ready for change.

Antabuse: Less common than it once was, this medication will make you violently ill with severe vomiting if you drink while on this medication. This is intended to be prophylactic motivation not to take a drink.

Suboxone: This is another opiate antagonist, also known as a *blocker*; however, it also contains an opiate, so it has high potential for its own abuse or addiction. This is not an ideal treatment if the goal is to be substance free. It is only used in patients who are dependent on short-acting opioids (e.g. heroin) and not for those on long-acting opioids (e.g. methadone). You don't need to go to a designated clinic for this, and it can be received from and monitored by your healthcare provider.

Methadone: This is used to treat opioid use disorder but is also a designated treatment for pain. It is a long-acting opioid antagonist that can blunt or block the effects of opioids. You can only get methadone from a designated methadone clinic. This has high potential for misuse and abuse and that can keep you chained to a drug.

Narcan: An opioid reversal agent. It is only used to reverse the effects of an opioid overdose. This is typically used by EMS, and now parents or other loved ones, to revive the patient.

Nonmedicinal treatments

Biofeedback: Biofeedback therapy is a non-drug treatment in which patients learn to control bodily processes that are normally involuntary, such as muscle tension, blood pressure, or heart rate. This is done by connecting painless electrodes to various places on the scalp. This analyzes and reports brain activity, and viewing this data, the person can alter breathing or make other changes to realign themselves. It's like putting things back in order for more homeostatic function of the brain. Biofeedback is used in training athletes as well as astronauts, but it's also used as an adjunct treatment for sleep disorder, ADHD, migraines, and a host of other medical conditions, such as addiction. Some say there is significant benefit in the treatment of addiction. One or more addiction treatment centers have been using this therapy with good results.

Transcranial Magnetic Stimulation: More specifically, *Theta Burst Magnetic Stimulation* (TBS), is another noninvasive therapy. It is a form of brain stimulation that more closely mimics the natural rhythms of activity in the neurons of the brain. Theta Bursts are short bursts of stimulation at high frequencies, with the bursts themselves being applied at a rate of five times per second. This uses magnetic fields to stimulate nerve cells in the brain to improve symptoms of depression. It's typically used when other treatments for depression have been unsuccessful. Some medical insurances cover TMS.

Ketamine IV Infusion Therapy: This may be a more controversial treatment option; however, it has been transformative for some individuals. Ketamine is an anesthetic currently used in the operating room. It is not currently FDA approved in IV infusion therapy for the treatment of depression, pain, and other mental health disorders. It is also not considered first-line treatment for these disorders. It does, however, have the potential to rapidly reduce suicidality and relieve other serious depressive symptoms. The FDA approved a nasal spray formulation of Ketamine for the treatment of depression in 2019.

Eye Movement Desensitization and Reprocessing (EMDR): This is a type of psychotherapy to treat trauma/PTSD and help relieve emotional distress through recalling troubling images and then redirecting eye movement. The goal is to help guide the brain to adaptive healing of the traumatic event. One website effectively describes it as "a way to get past your past."

Meditation: Meditation is an ancient practice that has been proven time and time again to effectively reduce stress, to ease anxiety and depression, to reduce blood pressure and heart rate, and to improve overall mood, concentration, and contentment. There is a mound of evidence supporting the use of meditation to improve overall health and, specifically, addiction. It is a technique regularly used in recovery. It involves sitting in quiet and stillness while relaxing the mind and body and directing one's attention away from distractions.

Group Therapy: Helpful groups may be virtual or in person, including AA, Smart Recovery, In the Room app, YouTube, and Facebook groups. If your loved one can't find a group, they simply aren't looking because one may attend them in person, find them online, or even just sit and listen without anyone knowing they are there. Groups can be found in every community coast to coast and now internationally online.

Online resources: There are about a million resources now, but one of my favorites, as I mention elsewhere, is *Put the Shovel Down* on Facebook. YouTube has so many motivators through their own channels or on Ted Talks. It's a matter of typing in keywords in a search field, and with just that, a whole other world can open up for your loved one.

FOR YOU:

As you might imagine, many of the exact same resources can be utilized by you. You're the other side of the coin in this, so it makes sense that you would use the same help lines.

Group Therapy

You may likely already know about Al-Anon and Nar-Anon, both globally accepted support groups for families of alcohol and substance use disorders, but there are other resources.

SMART Recovery: In person and online

Thrive Family Support: thrivefamilyrecoveryresources.org/support

In the Room: Phone app that lets you connect worldwide

CoDA: Codependents Anonymous, in person and online

Addiction Recovery Resources – Hope for Families: Support group on Facebook

Moms of Adult Addicts: Support group on Facebook

GRASP: Grief Recovery After Substance Passing. grasphelp.org

PAL: Parents of Addicted Loved Ones. palgroup.org

NAMI: National Alliance on Mental Illness. They provide advocacy, education, support, and public awareness, so all individuals and families affected by mental illness can build better lives. NAMI was the organization that helped me when my son was treated the way he was the night he was suicidal. I am eternally grateful for their assistance during one of the most difficult times in our lives.

Family Recovery Coach: Coaching is an incredible resource, and coaches help those affected by the addiction and recovery of another through their own recovery process.

State-Specific Help

Some resources are regional specific. I've listed a few from my area, but resources such as these are likely available for your region as well.

FAVOR: Faces and Voices of Recovery. Specific to South Carolina, but online nationwide.

Trillium Health Resources: For patients with serious substance use disorder, mental illness, and intellectual or developmental disabilities and for their loved ones. Specific to North Carolina.

OASAS: Office of Addiction Services and Supports. New York. oasas.ny.gov

Books That Saved Me

This is not an exhaustive list, and by no means are these the only resources in a sea of available books, but they are what fell into my life. I believe books come to you exactly when they are supposed to, and these did just that.

A Common Struggle: A Personal Journey Through the Past and Future of Mental Illness and Addiction, by Patrick J. Kennedy, Stephen Fried (Blue Rider Press, 2016).

Beautiful Boy: A Father's Journey Through His Son's Addiction, by David Sheff (Mariner Books, 2009).

The Big Book: Alcoholics Anonymous, by Bill W. (Alcoholics Anonymous World Services, Inc. Fourth Edition, 2002).

The Brain that Changes Itself: Stories of Personal Triumph From the Frontiers of Brain Science, by Norman Doidge (Viking, 2007).

Change Your Brain, Change Your Life: The Breakthrough Program for Conquering Anxiety, Depression, Obsessiveness, Lack of Focus, Anger, and Memory Problems, by Daniel G. Amen (Harmony, 2015).

Chasing the Scream: The Inspiration for the Feature Film "The United States vs. Billie Holiday," by Johann Hari (Bloomsbury USA, 2016).

Codependent No More: How to Stop Controlling Others and Start Caring for Yourself, by Melody Beattie (Hazelden, 1986).

Dream Seller: An Addiction Memoir, by Brandon Novak (Citadel, 2017).

Ego Is the Enemy, by Ryan Holiday (Portfolio, 2016).

The Five People You Meet in Heaven, by Mitch Albom (Hachette Books, 2003).

From Dope to Hope: A Man in Recovery, by Tim Ryan (Spiritus Communications, 2017).

GUTS: The Endless Follies and Tiny Triumphs of a Giant Disaster, by Kristen Johnston (Gallery Books, 2013).

The Last Lecture, by Randy Pausch, Jeffrey Zaslow (Hyperion, 2008).

Never Enough: The Neuroscience and Experience of Addiction, by Judith Grisel (Doubleday, 2019).

Saving Jake: When Addiction Hits Home, by D'Anne Burwell (FocusUp Books, 2015)

Recovery: Freedom From Our Addictions, by Russell Brand (Picador Paper, 2019).

Reinventing Your Life: The Breakthrough Program to End Negative Behavior and Feel Great Again, by Jeffrey E. Young, Janet S. Klosko, Aaron T. Beck (Plume, 1994).

The Shack: Where Tragedy Confronts Eternity, by William Paul Young (Windblown Media, 2007).

The Son I Knew Too Late: A Guide to Help You Survive and Thrive, by Sally A. Raymond (Sally A. Raymond, 2020).

Solve for Happy: Engineer Your Path to Joy, by Mo Gawdat (Gallery Books, 2018).

Ten Percent Happier: How I Tamed the Voice in My Head, Reduced Stress Without Losing My Edge, and Found Self-Help That Actually Works—A True Story, by Dan Harris (Dey Street Books, 2019).

Tweak: Growing Up on Methamphetamines, by Nic Sheff (Atheneum Books for Young Readers, 2009).

Unbroken Brain: A Revolutionary New Way of Understanding Addiction, by Maia Szalavitz (Picador, 2017).

Waking the Tiger: Healing Trauma, by Peter A. Levine, Ann Frederick (North Atlantic Books, 1997).

We Are the Luckiest: The Surprising Magic of a Sober Life, by Laura McKowen (New World Library, 2022).

What Happened to You? Conversations on Trauma, Resilience, and Healing, by Bruce D. Perry, Oprah Winfrey (Flatiron Books, 2021).

Your Brain Is Always Listening: Tame the Hidden Dragons That Control Your Happiness, Habits, and Hang-Ups, by Daniel G. Amen (Tyndale Refresh, 2021).

Podcasts That Spoke to Me

Unlocking Us, Brené Brown

Brandon Novak

Ted Radio Hour

Oprah's Super Soul Sunday and *20 Minutes for the Next 20 Years of Your Life*, Oprah

Controlling Everything? Here's How to Let Go and Trust the Universe, Dear Gabby

Addiction and the Family, Casey Arrillaga

Avoiding the Addiction Affliction, Mike McGowan

The Way Out, Charles LeVoir

My Steps to Sobriety, Dr. Stephan Neff

The Intentional Clinician, Paul Krauss MA LPC

YouTube Videos That Taught Me Something New

Put the Shovel Down, Amber Hollingsworth

CG Kid, Philip Markoff

The Elephant, The Rider, and The Path – A Tale of Behavior Change

23 ½ hours

National Hotlines

RAINN: National Sexual Assault Hotline 800-656-HOPE (4673), rainn.org

National Suicide Prevention Hotline: 800-273-TALK (8255), suicidepreventionlifeline.org

SAMHSA: Substance Abuse and Mental Health Service Administration, samhsa.gov

National Helpline (treatment referral and information) 800-662-HELP (4357)

NAMI: National Alliance on Mental Illness, 800-950-6264; or in crisis, text NAMI to 741741 for free crisis counseling

Talkspace.com

Additional Vocabulary

Until you're immersed in a foreign country for several years, you probably can't understand much of what anyone is saying. I've provided a short list of substance-related terminology I thought may be helpful, especially for those just hearing these terms for the first time. These are not Webster's Dictionary definitions; they are real-world definitions of experience as it is related to substance use disorders.

Active addiction: current abuse of a substance causing disruption of daily life and expectations. This is typically when individuals around those who are using substances feel the most out of control.

The word *addiction* itself has associated slang that you may overhear, such as *bent, hooked, monkey on your back, strung out, bagged.*

De-escalating: Calmly communicating with an agitated individual in order to understand, manage and resolve their concerns without major conflict. This may be in an effort to avoid a harmful situation.

Dry drunk: This describes an alcoholic who no longer drinks, but otherwise maintains the same behavior patterns of an alcoholic. In other words, a person may have quit drinking, but they have yet to deal with the emotional baggage that led them to alcohol in the first place. Dry drunk can be a volatile place to be because if the underlying issues aren't dealt with, there is a much higher chance of relapse.

Enabling: Providing the means, whether financial, emotional, or providing shelter, as examples, for a person to be able to continue their substance use without consequences.

Hospital or *rehab in-services:* In recovery, groups will collectively go to individuals in the hospital or other rehabs to provide information and hope for recovery. It may seem that this would only be helpful to the individuals receiving the in-services, however it can be even more helpful to those giving it as you learn to help others through the process.

Jonesing: Extreme desire for the addictive substance. It's like wanting to breathe air in some cases.

Pink cloud: This is a common phenomenon in individuals who are newly sober. It is characterized by feelings of elation, excitement, and a "ready to take on the world" attitude. Also called a *natural high* or a *honeymoon phase* in recovery. It can last for days to weeks but can have negative effects when it wears off and reality sets in.

Relapse: The recurrence of substance use disorder or use in any person who has gone into remission or recovery.

A person who *sells* drugs to your loved one may be called *pill lady, pump, source, pusher, mad hatter, middleman.*

Sponsor: In AA, this is essentially your mentor, coach, and counselor to get you through the everyday and the toughest moments. They are always available on the other end of the phone or in person when you need someone to get you through a craving or life in general.

Under the influence is referred to as *baked, blazed, burned, caramelized, crossfaded, crunched, crunk, dankrupt, faded, geeked, hurt, keyed, krunked, lifted, lit, skunt, sloppy, smoked, stuck, zoned.*

Withdrawal: Symptoms such as sweating, uncontrollable tremors, inability to sleep, agitation, and even seizures, heart attack, or sudden death when a person abruptly stops using drugs or alcohol after prolonged and excessive use.

I encourage an internet search on slang terms directly related to your loved one's DOC or drug of choice. There are extensive lists related to the individual drugs and related paraphernalia. The best resource I found was at recoveryanswers.org/addiction-ary/.

I wish I could say this covers it all, but in reality, it is not even close. I did not know these associations, websites, groups, or words existed when this all came rushing into our lives, but they are all available to you when you're ready to use them.

CHAPTER 20

MENTAL HEALTH

We rise by lifting others.
~ often attributed to Robert Ingersoll

It takes ten years, on average, to make the diagnosis of bipolar disorder. It is an elusive condition that can be very difficult to tease out of a myriad of mental health possibilities. It can mimic drug intoxications, brain tumors, endocrine disorders, head trauma, PTSD, or even the consequences of sleep deprivation. It is characterized by episodes lasting weeks to months of alternating and debilitating mania and depression.

My son has never had a manic event. *Mania* can include staying awake for days at a time, emptying out your bank account, suddenly thinking you can do things you've never done before, like run for president. Grandiose thinking can best describe someone with bipolar I disorder, but there is also a type II. *Hypomania* is the type of elevated state exhibited in bipolar II disorder and is defined by a more subdued elation followed by severe depressive episodes.

In late 2021, after four blissful months of sobriety, my son went from an elated level of happiness I had not seen since he was a child to a chaotic storm of emotions that plunged him into a deep depression in less than twenty-four hours. The pandemonium that ensued took on a whole new level of illness.

My son was facing an adventure and moving west to Arizona with his girlfriend. Kate was starting a new job, and Tyler had just passed the test for his commercial drone licensure. He was ready to ask Kate to marry him and to start their journey together to explore new destinations and take on new adventures.

Self-sabotage is a common phenomenon known to those with substance use disorder. Just when things are at their very best, and you have absolutely everything you could ever want, you take a nose dive with your DOC and step out of life for whatever amount of time it takes to recognize what has happened. Many will say the reasoning is that those with the disease of addiction combined with a mental health condition, like depression, have an underlying belief that they truly don't deserve the positive things coming to them in their life. Others recognize stress, even positive stress, can be a trigger for relapse. As the parent watching this, I can tell you self-sabotage can sometimes be more heartbreaking than addiction itself. To see the potential and then to see it fade away is like trying to hug a ghost—you feel the presence, but as soon as you get too close, it evaporates.

Tyler and Kate left with two weeks to explore the country on their way to their new destination. However, within a few short hours, the adventure turned dark, and Tyler started drinking: six bottles of wine each day, after being sober for four months. He lost all control and experienced something called *alcohol-induced psychosis*. He turned into the Hyde version of Jekyll and Hyde—and completely disassociated with reality due to alcohol alone. The police were called three times in a week for crisis intervention. They brought him to the hospital one time, but he ran before they could do an assessment.

The third intervention was in New Mexico. In this state, if the police are called for any reason, the person at the heart of the conflict will be taken out of the current scene and be put in jail. So, he detoxed in a jail once again, but somehow his faculties returned to baseline, and he became coherent and somewhat aware of his actions.

Alex and I were stranded in North Carolina. We were getting calls from Kate, who was in the same state of mind I had been in for the more-than ten years prior: distraught, crying, confused, hurt, angry, and sad. Her whole life was imploding right before her, and her job in Arizona was on the line. We did what we could to console her and attempted to talk to Tyler when he would have rare episodes of awareness. We also talked with the officers to try to help, but it all seemed fruitless from where we were sitting.

This time, however, was different. We didn't get sucked in to the black hole of despair like we had so many times before. We were much more rational and reserved. Don't get me wrong: I had moments of pulling my hair out and spells of crying, but I refused to fall into the well with him this time. I wouldn't be of any use there. My husband and I worked together in the same camp to figure out some semblance of a plan for Tyler, whereas before, we were in the same universe but sometimes on opposite ends of it.

While Tyler slept in jail, we methodically looked up rehab options for him to try one more time. We at least knew he was safe, in the most generous sense of the word, and most certainly unable to use any alcohol. The key here was that Alex and I did this research together. Not that we hadn't in the past, but the decision-making and phone calls had fallen mostly on my shoulders. This time he made multiple phone calls, talked to the officers and rehab intake counselors and, with a highly organized effort, reviewed the options.

We even put together a spreadsheet to compare the options before us:

CENTER	LOCATION	JCAHO	INDVIDUAL COUNSELING	EMDR	12-STEP	Dual DX	OTHER
Sample Recovery	Laos, NM	Yes	Once wkly	Yes	No	Yes	505-436-****
Sample Healing Center	Scottsdale, AZ	No	Once wkly	Yes	Yes	Yes	480-825-**** Cole
Sample Center	Scottsdale, AZ	Yes	Twice wkly	Yes	No/ SMART	Yes	602-668-****

When I cried, Alex took care of me and the task before us. He made plane reservations and, within twelve hours, was flying out to pick Tyler up from jail to take him to rehab.

Should we have helped him again? I have no idea. There will never be a road map. There will never be a perfect plan, and there will never be a right answer at the right time. You have to listen to your instincts. I felt that we could show him the opportunity, but he would be on his own if he chose not to take it. We would not enable, but we would help facilitate.

I will never say a crisis experience gets easy or is perfectly manageable, but we approach it differently now and with much more level heads. This is something I wish I had been able to conquer many years before. I honestly can't even believe I can talk about a crisis experience as if it were something normal, because it isn't—but it is our reality and we needed to be armed and ready instead of caught off guard and left in the fetal position in the closet, as I had been.

My son still does not have a mental health diagnosis, and we still have no real idea if this episode was triggered by that or by something else entirely. Tyler is a picture of the perfect storm. Substance abuse and mental health genetics, divorce, initiating alcohol use at age twelve, bullying, lack of social support, and trauma. Regardless of our dilemma, I felt it was an important subject to cover due to the known high incidence of correlating mental health and SUD. It is crucial to figure out whether mental health is part of the picture.

My son has remained in remission since that last episode. He was able to work with some of the best, most responsive and respectful therapists he had seen up to that point. They were the first to change his perspective. I could hear it in his words and more importantly, see it in his actions each and every day.

One day, Tyler actually said, "I'm glad I have such a severe form of this condition because I can't ever fool myself into thinking that I am somehow functional despite my excessive alcohol use."

Only a healthy mind could come to that conclusion.

CHAPTER 21

FAMILY LIES

"Forgiveness is healing." He smiles. "Especially forgiving yourself."
~ Alyson Noel
Evermore

Every family member has their preconceived opinions and understanding—or lack of them, in many cases—about your addicted loved one. It can come from lack of education, but if you told them your child or significant other had cancer, they would rally around you, support you, listen to your every word, and wrap you in their warmth.

When you tell them your child or other loved one has an addiction, family members' opinions and judgments can come spewing out of them as if they know everything there is to know about this elusive disease. Their opinions are sometimes hurtful, cold, and cruel. This is why we isolate, hide, and tell lies to cover up what is happening in our homes. I truly do love my family, but as with most families, that comes with multidimensional issues and unresolved resentments.

When the family would get together, we'd always got to this point of contention about drinking while my son was there. It seemed fairly simple to me, in my rationalizing mind, that you just shouldn't drink alcohol in his presence until he verbalized that he was alright with it. If I were out with a friend and they were newly diagnosed with diabetes, would I order an ice cream cone and lick the drippings off my hand while moaning about the deliciousness of it in front of them? Would I order the largest piece of chocolate cake at a restaurant when I'm out with a family member that is desperately trying to lose weight? Never. I'd like to call it *conscientiousness*.

And yet when it's suggested to hold on the alcohol consumption at a family gathering or other event, some people seem almost indignant—like I took away their soothing pacifier. *Why should I not be able to drink when I'm not the one with the problem? Why can't they just deal with it and get it together, so I don't have to be put out if only for a few mere hours of abstinence?* However, I can also see that when we restrict supply, we might ignite the desire for even more, in the same way you want chocolate cake even more when you're trying to avoid it. It's likely best to let the person with the disease guide the rest of us to make the right decisions at the right time, but as any of us who have tried to have that conversation know, it can be difficult.

So often, immediate family members, admittedly me to begin with, fail to do the aforementioned education. We disconnect and avoid and tell lies to keep the peace, to deflect, to hide—just like the addict. So, if the opportunity presents itself and it's the right time, I suggest you try like hell to put it all out there.

Those who love you will always show up and do what's right and be helpful. And if they don't, first try to educate. Then, cut your losses for the time being, if only to save yourself. It took about seven years, after we fully understood what was happening, for me to start telling people. At first, I found it most rewarding to share with my patients, who were also struggling with the same experiences. It came naturally. Who better to reveal your soul to than those already living your nightmare? I later found the courage to stand up and give speeches and put all the ugliness on display for the very people I felt were globally responsible for my son's decline. And finally, after conceding for too long, I was able to reveal the truth to my closest family and friends.

As time goes on, you might battle with the resentments you feel toward your family for their blind participation or lack of awareness and involvement, but you have to ask yourself: *Could my resentment actually be a mirror of myself?* My family, who lived in the same city as my son, drank with him often. After the realization of the severity of his illness, I was angry with them, and I failed to accept their lack of understanding. Truthfully, they were duped as much as I was, but I thought they should have been able to see better because they were so up close and personal. It was all an effort to shift the blame and not look directly in the eye of the problem.

There can be months and years of misunderstandings and resentments that develop in your families. This can work against getting any kind of serious help for your loved one. Being a unified force when fighting this disease is crucial. I made at least a thousand mistakes with my son and was able to admit that, but it is just as important for everyone else to recognize their part.

My sister, for example, *has a heart of gold*, which is something people often say right before revealing a hard truth. She truly only sees the good in people, forgiving them of things no one else would even think about forgiving. After years of her denying my son's true depth of affliction, I accumulated so much resentment. I often felt that because she remained so functional in her own substance use, she simply assumed my son could. Or maybe he lied to her as eloquently as he did with me, convincing her he was just fine, but while my son lived with her, she would drink with him on a regular basis. She saw him at his worst and never called to make me aware of anything. He was drowning and she was pulling him under. It's difficult to reconcile because I love my sister, and I know the trauma she has experienced. I've always cut her a break because of it, but when it affected my child, not herself alone, it felt like it went too far.

I also understood addiction and its far-reaching effects, so I had to extend that understanding to her and not just to my son. I have empathy for my son, my patients, and all individuals with this disease, so why wouldn't I have that same understanding with my sister's addictions? The truth is I do, but her addiction caused her to cross a boundary with my son, which is desperately hard to resolve emotionally. I've had to figure out a way to separate the two. I've had to compartmentalize so many feelings all just to make it through this.

If my sister was an enabler, then my mother was an avoider. They both maintain a firm grasp on the idea that if they can do something, then everyone else should be able to figure it out as well. Which, of course, is not at all realistic. So, I believe they felt he should just be able to *get over it*—to overcome it and just figure his shit out.

My mom could not comprehend the magnitude of the problem. Most of the time, she would pretend it simply didn't exist. And she, too, drank with my son, but in her defense, Tyler was exceptional at hiding his addiction from her as well. He could drink a beer or two with her and pretend he didn't want any more, but then he would leave and be blacked out before the night was over. I tried to tell her, and his dad and my sister, and so many others, but no one could really grasp what I was saying—or maybe it was just easier to disassociate.

Addicts are non-malicious manipulators and deceivers, and they get very good at their craft. Tyler, on the other hand, was boldly honest with me, which left me with information no one else could know. It was maddening. Even Alex wasn't fully aware of the depth of the issue for many years. Despite Tyler's multiple DUIs, multiple rehabs, and multiple legal issues, my closest family members remained in disbelief. People tended to just look away and chalk it up to youth or stupidity. I was in that same headspace for many years, so how could I blame them? Unfortunately, families can be unintentional enablers.

It wasn't until the gastric bleed and the hospitalizations for pancreatitis that friends and family started recognizing how serious the problem was. All of a sudden, I got phone calls from far-away friends and family who finally became aware they could lose Tyler to this disease. Their tears were enough to fill buckets, but I had been crying oceans for ten years. Where had these people been all along? And then when the trauma was revealed, the whole world seemed to give him, and me for helping him, a break.

I came to accept that we have to rely on our families and be honest with them because their help can be lifesaving to us and our addicted loved ones. If you don't have family support in any way, then your foundation will not be able to withstand the addiction experience. That may be a bold assertion, but as they say, it does take a village.

The village may need to be found elsewhere—with friends, in the church of your choosing, or support groups. Basically, what I am saying is: Don't try to go it alone. The person with substance use disorder is told the same thing: Never isolate. It's not an option for us, either, because no matter what, you will need help, so find your village.

I will add that if our society had better universal education, understanding, legislation, and legal and medical intervention, this overwhelming issue would improve. But isn't that the case with most situations? We all focus on what matters most to us personally. This disease simply doesn't affect all of us. With so many issues in the world, it has become increasingly difficult to evoke any change despite the critical need for it. Socially and culturally, we are just not there yet. And yet ironically, an overwhelming number of families are affected to some degree by this particular epidemic.

I had to remember that family is everything. It took a while to heal past my perceptions and to forgive. I love my mom and my sister, and they, just as I had to, did the best they could with what they knew at the time. They may not be perfect or always helpful, but when no one else showed up, they did. It may have been begrudgingly at times, yet they still tried.

You need your family. Help them to understand. Give them any resources you can find—I wish I had—but most of all, give them a break. Addiction is a universally misunderstood, mischaracterized, and sidestepped disease, even by those most affected by it.

For centuries, the *town drunk* or whatever wayward individual with substance use disorder or mental health issue in the family was not acknowledged or discussed; they were simply put away or institutionalized and completely forgotten about. While that is not acceptable treatment anymore, we still don't know how to effectively treat these beautiful people. Everyone with substance use disorder has a heart, a purpose, and a contribution. We all just have to be willing to be compassionate, listen, and give them the emotional support they desperately need.

The family unit is a crucial stabilizing force when a loved one is addicted. Many people may not live in an ideal situation in their current household, although I don't know if *an ideal situation* exists. I recognize my relationship with my husband was functional and resourceful. Working with him—and, to a small degree, with my ex-husband—nourished the real work of substance recovery. I also recognize I had medical, financial, and social education that clued me in to more information and resources. I will always be grateful for and clearly recognize the advantages we had.

CHAPTER 22

FACING FACEBOOK

Silence and reserve will give anyone a reputation for wisdom.
~ Myrtle Reed
Old Rose and Silver

It may be unusual to examine social media in a book about addiction, however there is a role that is played by this particular entity, and it's worth trying to understand. If you were to look me up on Facebook, it would appear that my life was blessed, easy, and free-spirited most of the time. What a façade social media is.

I went to Italy for the first time in my life while my son was sober. Our pictures on Facebook captured true joy, but it was only because of the context of our life at the time as it is for anyone, I suppose. The life we portrayed was rarely parallel to what we were experiencing, but appearances became more important than truth.

I've always been private—ironically so, considering I'm baring every corner of my soul here. There seems to be this tendency to put forward what appears simple and pleasant, maybe even contrived, in the world of social media. The key word, again, being *appears*. I didn't want to ruin anyone else's day with my problems. I didn't ask for prayers on social media or repost great quotes on overcoming addiction, although there are many. It occurred to me that seeing others' posts was affecting me in unpleasant ways, but it took me a while to fully understand why.

My mom had been swallowed whole by the political forcefield found on Facebook. We literally felt we lost her somewhere in the social media cosmos. Not to mention, Facebook was also the very platform used by the most unthinkable bully in my son's life—the one that told him to go kill himself. Facebook was the source that enabled this hate to transpire.

As a result of these experiences, my exposure became less and less, but somehow, I came across the awareness of Amber Hollingsworth through Facebook—another one of those divine interventions, I'd like to think. She's the first person who turned the counseling experience on its head for me. She answers the questions you don't even know you have or questions you simply don't know how to ask. She makes things make sense. Her YouTube channel was pivotal for me.

Even though I was seeing a therapist, our sessions at times felt like a lot of simply hearing myself talk. I know this can be hugely therapeutic, but sometimes you just want someone to tell you what to do. The YouTube channel *Put the Shovel Down* finally gave me clear and concise and actionable solutions. I needed her ten years ago, so hopefully you'll look her up much sooner than I did.

My husband and I had a presence on social media, but we essentially dropped out of life. Trying to explain decades of research to people with preconceived ideas of the disease of addiction was beyond daunting and out of the question. It became easier and easier to fade into the background than to say everything was always great and fine. It became uncomplicated to not see how perfect other people's children were, whether they really were or not. Looking at other families' amazing children on social media became exhausting. I was a decent mother who loved her child more than her own life, but I got handed the struggle. The truth of the matter was I was envious. I desperately wanted the ease I thought they had. Maybe they did something so much better than I did that their child didn't have to struggle. Or maybe social media is just an idealized projection of what we are trying to achieve.

It took me a full decade to release those foolish thoughts, and removing myself from so much social media helped. I saw parent after parent in my medical office with a brood of children, and inevitably one or more would have a struggle with mental health, substances, or something even worse. They would all be raised with the same amount of love and experiences that the other children had, but things turned out differently for some.

It wasn't what the parents had done in most cases, it was the result of many factors. Peers, society, trauma, multiple moves, genetics, losing friends, no relatives—the list can go on and on. I clawed through the Earth's mantle to figure out what I had done only to learn that I had done the very best I could with what I knew at that time. And, most importantly, I learned how compromising Facebook and other social media platforms can be. They all lack authenticity. I appreciated the superficiality of social media, but once it became a cancer of its own, even aimed at my own family, the value of it plummeted.

However, I had to accept that maybe, just maybe, there are positive attributes of social media.

As it turns out, I ended up finding some help with my own recovery from the very source I was trying to avoid. Not just with *Put the Shovel Down*, as previously mentioned, but I connected there with the <u>Family in Recovery</u> resource. For the first time, I wrote a revealing part of myself that I previously thought would be impossible to do, and it felt like I was invited to a public speaking engagement for the first time in my life. I was actually breaking down a very private wall to expose everything all at once. Apparently, it was the crack that broke the levy because it was soon after that when I began to write. I didn't say much really, but it was a pivotal experience. I guess Facebook showed me it had the potential to be an asset and not just a negative influence in our lives.

Hello everyone,

I'm new and trying to figure myself out in this messed up experience of my son's addiction. After ten years, many, many relapses, countless detoxes, sober livings, six rehabs, legal, medical, and financial consequences, I want to continue to examine myself and what my role has been in all of this.

My son is not the lying, stealing type. He's the brutally honest, here's-what-it-looks-like, feel-my-pain, forever-apologetic, suicidal, alone-in-his-vehicle-drinking-himself-into-oblivion type with underlying severe depression and debilitating anxiety—again, made so much worse with substance abuse.

Depression with the grand ignitor, alcohol, poured like gasoline on a fire. He's ridiculously knowledgeable in addiction, recovery, AA, psychology, and philosophy, seeing and knowing exactly what he is doing to himself and others while doing it. He can tell others exactly what it takes to be sober. He can tell himself exactly what he needs to do, do it, and still use. We have let him figure it out for years with no success or progression, and I can't find people with this same experience. What can I do differently in this situation?

I approach him with love, understanding of the disease, and compassion while trying not to enable. He's getting help from doctors and counselors, but it's not working. He states very clearly that he has no desire to use even when he's using. It's like a handicapped toddler who bangs their head against the wall even though it causes pain. None of this seems like the typical story, or maybe that's just my perception? What else can I do?

Regardless, thanks for reading. It's nice just to have found this resource.

This was the very first time I revealed what was happening to us, although I clearly wasn't yet being honest with myself about enabling my son. I didn't think I could be that vulnerable. In fact, I sat there for a very long time with my finger over the Post button. As it turned out, a lot of people responded to my post with thoughtful and helpful information. It was cathartic sharing, revealing, exposing. Pain cascaded out of my soul. This was another element that helped heal my relationship with myself.

What we see on these platforms is a tiny fraction of real existence. We must keep social media in perspective. It's not an indication of who we are, the life we are living, or the values we truly have, in most cases. Most importantly, don't let these images fool you into believing everything is okay. Behind the image is a real person who may be suffering.

CHAPTER 23

GREATER UNDERSTANDING

*Every morning we are born again.
What we do today is what matters most.*
~ Buddha

I once read that if you were not especially religious before your experience parenting a child with addiction, you will be after. I'm pretty sure I read that in another parent's memoir—no surprise. Religion is such an intimate and personal thing. When you throw in the hellfire that is addiction, it can cause you to examine your internal relationship with faith more closely. I know some of you who are walking with addiction in your family have figured it out much more than I have. I know others who have been able to lay this all down from the very beginning and walk away on nothing but faith. I was not one of them. I was too analytical and demanding—or stubborn, some may also say—not to discover what I thought should be mere mortal solutions to the disease of addiction and to saving my son. When this all began, I wasn't aware of my own need to be saved.

It felt ironic to try to find faith when I was in crisis, overwhelmingly confused and furious at the very source who was supposed to bring me peace and solace. I had to come face to face with the God of my understanding through this daunting experience. Never mind that I had never felt exactly religious. I have, however, always been spiritual. Spirituality seemed to come with some essence of freedom and room to make mistakes without the overriding and irrational fear of eternal damnation. Ultimately, for me, faith had to become the ability to stop looking for answers. I had to find the faith to capture patience and peace. My understanding of faith eventually became giving up control, living for today, and simply being grateful for another day with my son.

But it took so much to get there. In this experience, we become scavengers, looking for faith and peace anywhere we can possibly find it. It becomes an endless struggle to hold on just one more day. I would have walked to the ends of the Earth if the answers had been there. So many times, I tried to tell myself that I could simply turn away from my understanding of God. I felt so betrayed and abandoned, and I just couldn't accept what I was facing—what my son was facing. Why would a loving God allow us all to hurt this badly for this long?

In the midst of the mental turmoil, I stopped fighting and questioning, and I started listening and understanding. I began to see the big picture and the interconnectedness these experiences really provided. I experienced the coincidences—some would say *miracles*—that had no other viable explanation. I had to step out of the bubble we were in and look at it from a different vantage point to understand the complexity. As a result, I began to understand things more dimensionally. I realized then it was only fair to contribute my understanding to the same force I was accusing of taking my light away.

When the COVID-19 pandemic happened, and they started talking about the shedding of viral particles, I realized, on a more introspective level, that this is exactly what each of us is doing every second of every day with every word, movement, or breath. We're all essentially shedding life particles or particles of ourselves—some would call *energy*—that never leave. These particles accumulate like metaphysical residue. I needed this understanding to handle my son's reality—that he may be swallowed whole by this disease—and to comprehend that we all really live forever.

This led me to the understanding of my son's contribution as well as my own. He touched so many lives because of his illness. I came to understand that his existence transcends his life. We never really die because our residue is always left behind. This enlightenment kept me walking through the constant maze we were in and helped me to see that we exist through connection—that we are so much more than the 100 or so years we are given.

As difficult as it is to admit this, it also helped me to come to terms with the possibility of actually losing my son. This holds us captive to their addiction: They can die from this, and we can lose them forever. It doesn't mean we are giving up, but acknowledging this irrefutable truth can allow us to let go. I have had the gift of learning so much from Tyler. He has given me understanding that never would have occurred otherwise. He's done that for others too.

This understanding helped me to reflect on my son's contributions and not his disease or his mistakes alone.

The experience of addiction as a whole can be so much bigger than we let ourselves realize. I learned who my son was through this tragedy. He is a humanitarian in the truest sense of the word. He's always had a profound globalized awareness of pain. We're all aware of genocide, global hunger, plastic in our oceans, and human trafficking, but this awareness typically doesn't influence our daily thoughts or actions. We're not profoundly crushed by the weight of that knowledge like some are. Like my son was at times.

My sweet child would sit on the sidewalk with a homeless person for hours and just talk. He had no judgment or fear of those situations. To this day, he won't even kill a spider. When he sits down to eat, he thanks the animal that gave its life so that he can have sustenance, every time.

There were several years when the disease took more hold of him, and he became more detached—never violent or mean, but rarely content. He had pounded down his serotonin with the alcohol hammer so many times, it had almost no hope of rebounding. He had stopped being that compassionate and aware human because he couldn't do anything about the pain of the world, so he just carried it and became solemn and unattached. It was a transition that was brutal to witness. Knowing the gleeful, glowing child and seeing his eyes full of despair was surely hell. I later understood that it wasn't just the weight of the world that had stolen his joy. It was a real-life monster who tried to take the light from his eyes.

We all seem to take on our understanding of faith at one point or another. Sometimes we're simply raised to understand faith from one perspective only, and that can certainly be a source of hope and comfort. But when you're confronted with this agonizing disease, it can make you question everything you thought you always knew. It puts you in conflict with yourself and your understanding of God. It makes you want to give up on the idea of faith. You pray and pray and pray and ask why your prayers aren't being answered. You give up on prayers and on the God of your understanding. But that doesn't work either.

Telling someone how to face their religion during this tumultuous time is like trying to tell your addicted loved one to simply stop using. I equate it to climbing my personal Mount Everest. I just couldn't accept that I wasn't the one in control, but when I finally relinquished it, my soul felt washed.

When you pay attention to the events in your life or in the life of your addicted loved one, you may see things that can't be explained by words alone. There have been too many miracles of coincidence. Finding my son in his hidden car when he was suicidal was the least of them. The very words you are reading have appeared in an other-worldly way. I can't begin to explain where my time or ability to formulate these words and thoughts came from or how I even found the courage to share this with those who may need it most.

If you pray for the right people to come into your life and your loved one's, the right people at the right time may just show up. Or if you thank the God of your understanding for another day, you simply get another day, and what is more wonderous than that? We will never know how this experience is designed for us, but we have to trust our faith when absolutely nothing else makes any sense, when we're down on the floor, drowning in a puddle of our own tears, screaming out for their survival and for our own.

Even as my son has come face to face with the devil, I choose to remain connected spiritually because I know there will be a crown of glory for him someday. If you force yourself to confront your understanding of faith while holding on for dear life to anything that makes sense, then you are doing it right. You are doing the best you can. Whatever faith looks like in your world, I hope you will lean into it, fall into it, and let go.

CHAPTER 24

LESSONS LEARNED

You can't wait until life isn't hard anymore before you decide to be happy.
~ Jane Marczewski

It was that glorious day in March of 2021 when I let go and began to heal. Nothing remarkable ignited the transformation. It was probably the accumulation of repeatedly hearing words like *natural consequences* and *setting boundaries*, but also the painful realization that I had become addicted to the frenzied illusion of control over my addicted loved one. Maybe it was all the writing that set me free. My focus shifted—oddly as it seems, since I'm writing about him for the most part—from him to everything else.

Lesson One: Allow Yourself to Let Go

As we age, we're supposed to accumulate life lessons. I went about it the hard way, resisting at the very times I should have been listening, but when I let go, I also stopped resisting. I started listening to those voices around me I had tried to tune out. But most importantly, I started paying attention to the many lessons I had gathered. My sincere hope is that these lessons reach you earlier in your quest for answers rather than later.

I found personal insight in many places. My husband has always been a man of few words, but when he formulates them, they are typically spot on and noteworthy. He once said, "Every mom of a police officer, military professional, or a cancer patient has the constant fear of their child's death in the back of their mind." It made me realize I am not alone in feeling crippling fear of my child's potential death. That knowledge also made me feel less broken.

He also said, "Do you really think *exceptional parenting* had the power to overcome genetics, normal teenage experience, and the assault our son experienced? Did you think you had that much influence?" He wasn't being critical; he was making practical sense.

I never really thought I was an exceptional parent, but I also never felt like I failed completely. I did what every parent believes is right in the moment. This insight didn't mean I stopped worrying, but it meant I stopped letting his disease dictate my life. It gave me clarity.

Lesson Two: Create Connections

I discovered the unmatched value of connection. Just knowing the battles that other families routinely faced gave me a sense of common ground. In the practice of medicine, you are up-close and personal with others' lives. I empathetically connected with so many mothers and fathers because of my chosen career, and I am grateful for that. We suffered together instead of in silence. That can breathe hope into life.

At some point, I did learn to write down the name of every doctor, friend, counselor, and dealer, and to record house addresses and place of employment related to my son. This gave me peace of mind at times because I had an imaginary link to him, even if it wasn't directly with him. If someone called me, I immediately saved their number. Mothers of friends, friends of friends, lawyers—it didn't matter.

Now, I don't know if this is exactly a positive discovery or something you'd want to adopt because, let's be honest, it feeds into your addiction, but there are times it saved my son's life. So many of these people helped save me as well. They gave me hope and words of encouragement when I needed to hear them, and they reminded me how wonderful my son was. Tyler has been truly loved and admired by so many people along his sordid path.

Maintaining these contacts didn't exactly leave room for natural consequences, but sometimes you have to do what is right based solely on your gut.

Lesson Three: You Can't Do It for Them

The discovery for an answer to my eternal search for what was enabling and what wasn't formed after a long time:

- If you pay their rent, or phone bill, or for groceries so that they can continue to buy their drug of choice, you are enabling.
- If you give them a roof over their head so they don't have to thrive independently, then you are enabling.
- If you get them out of jail or pay their legal fees, then you are enabling.
- If you buy them cars or pay for repeated repairs, then once again, you are enabling.

I feel like everyone knows these things logically, but the parents I see in my practice continue to find stealthy ways to enable their loved ones while justifying their actions out of love and fear, just like I did. And sometimes just hearing or reading the simplest things makes that part of your brain return to logic and realize what you're doing. You simply can't recover *for* your loved one—trust me, I tried and tried. You can encourage, and you can remind them that they are loved, but you cannot provide the means for them to continue their use.

It seems ludicrous today that I couldn't fully grasp the concept of how I was enabling my son, but I always asked myself: *If he had cancer, what would I be doing?* And the answer is, if he had cancer, I would stop at nothing to help him survive—so why wouldn't I do the same for this disease?

I had to accept this wasn't cancer. It is too socially, emotionally, and medically different to be viewed in the same vein. The answer, I decided for myself, is to let them know you love them with all your heart, you will never abandon them, and you will be there to help them in any way you're able while supporting their sobriety. But you can't do it for them. Give them the knowledge that you believe they can do it. And pray.

Lesson Four: Understand How You Are Enabling

I stopped asking God for what I so desperately wanted and simply thanked him for another day with my son. If he was sober, I thanked God for his sobriety that day.

I had to discover for myself when to shut up. Imagine someone repeatedly saying:

I don't want you to live your life the way you're living it.
I don't want you to live your life the way you're living it.
I don't want you to live your life the way you're living it.
I don't want you to live your life the way you're living it.

How many times can you read that before becoming annoyed? This is what we do to addicts because, seriously, we don't want them to live the way they are! As hard as it was, I had to learn to allow him to live his life the way *he* wanted to. It wasn't the way I wanted him to choose to live, but I had to accept that I didn't get to decide that for another adult. I am not deaf to the dilemma that letting them live their lives can also mean they might die as a result of the way they are living it. Therein lies the very core of the issue. Letting go versus not letting go is the toughest choice you will face in this whole experience.

I am not suggesting you stand aside and let your loved one harm themselves; you must work through your choices. Learn to effectively communicate with your loved one so it is productive and not argumentative. Educate yourself so that you are fully equipped when opportunities arrive for discussion. Accept them for exactly who they are. Meeting people where they are means accepting without bringing your judgment to their story. Listen to your loved one to understand and not necessarily to respond.

Lesson Five: Accept That You Can Release Your Addicted Loved One

Some kids want parental handholding, but that was definitely not the case for my son. My son came into this world under duress. He had the nuchal cord wrapped around his neck, and he was whisked away from me before I even got to see him. I had to wait for two days to hold my son for the first time. He became fiercely independent right out of the gate, but sometimes I don't think the cord was ever cut by me, by life, or by him. I had to learn to stop holding his hand by giving chronic advice. How annoying I'd become in my effort to be the savior of my son.

I've met many parents who have never gotten to the point of self-reckoning. I've even known some who have gone to their graves while still holding the rope on the edge of the cliff for their loved one. When finally arriving at the point of reason for yourself, it can be like running through the finish line ribbon at the end of a marathon. You'll be exhausted but elated, knowing you finally got smacked around enough not to take it anymore. You can love the individual with substance use disorder without existing through them. Accepting mortality—meaning we all have a time to live and a time to die, and we possess no control of time—offered me, at least, an ounce of peace and acceptance.

LESSONS LEARNED

Lesson Six: Do What Works

My son figured out how to make sobriety work during his two-year sober sabbatical in 2018, when the planets aligned, and he did absolutely everything imaginable to remain in remission:

- He surrounded himself with other sober people at all times.
- He went to meetings.
- He did hospital and rehab in-services.
- He participated in his own rehab alumni group.
- He exercised.
- He meditated.
- He got a job.
- He managed a sober living setting.
- He ate well.
- He prayed.
- He went to see a counselor every single week.
- He visited his PCP regularly.
- He socialized with other sober people.
- He had a sponsor whom he called almost daily.
- He slept on a regular schedule.
- He became a sponsor to others.

Remaining in remission became its own full-time job. It is no joke, and that's well known by individuals with this disorder. Our planets need to align as well to discover that we need to be as equally dedicated to our rebirth as they are to theirs.

I also discovered that writing and talking to a counselor after ten years of bottled-up anguish was transformative. It was the releasing of all the poison that had built up inside me for so long. Finding an outlet was crucial. I thought I was working it out by constantly ruminating. If I just sat quietly and thought through everything, wasn't I, in effect, working it out? Why did I need to talk to someone or write like I told my patients to do a thousand times? I needed to take the medicine I had so generously dispensed to others.

Lesson Seven: Release Yourself From Guilt and Judgment
I also learned that guilt became part of my disease. It needed to be cut out as badly as a cancerous tumor does.

I went through all the self-accusatory, ridiculous questions, including:
- Was the lack of oxygen or lack of my touch at birth a contributory factor to his addiction?
- Did the antibiotics that were given to him the day he was born cause his attention deficit disorder?
- Did I drink alcohol before I knew I was pregnant?
- Why didn't I evaluate the genetic history of my son's father before planning a family?
- Should I have moved him closer to family?
- Should I have put him in better schools?
- Did the divorce from his dad play a part or, even worse, is this what the outcome of a generation of divorces looks like?
- What did I do wrong?

Furthermore, I discovered most of us assume others are judging us or our loved ones, and that assumption is likely incorrect. The son of one of my patients had been in a wheelchair since the age of ten, when he had a tumor removed from his brain. He had no disability prior to that surgery, but he was never the same after. I took the time to inquire about him and ask how she has been able to handle his care all her life.

She told me that she never talked to anyone about her son except minimally with her sister. I asked her why. She sat there for a few minutes and said, "Well, I've never really thought about that." Then she started laughing a bit awkwardly toward herself and said after a pause, "I guess I want people to think he's doing better than he really is."

I've thought about that answer so much because I found myself doing the same thing when answering questions about my son. Are we protecting ourselves from judgment? Are we shielding our loved one from misperceptions? Why do we remain in such isolation?

There are those who judge everyone around them from the minute they're born until the day they die. Isn't it about time we recognize that as their problem, not ours? I have spoken openly in the medical practice about my son and found people to be receptive, understanding, and compassionate. So many people are carrying unspeakable burdens. Releasing those burdens without fear of judgment promotes both physical and mental healing. I'm not glad my son has had this affliction or that he's had to carry a burden he did not ask for, but I'm grateful for the experience of developing better understanding and acceptance of others. I accept people exactly as they are.

Lesson Eight: Resist Expectations and Assumptions

I also learned that everything boils down to our expectations. That frustrating definition of *a belief that someone will or should achieve something* defined the way I raised my son. I unwittingly had a one-track mind for my son's growth and life. I can't say I know exactly how that happened, but likely it was from generational expectations passed down to me. More than anything, I expected him to be accomplished, happy, and easy.

I got the very opposite, which made me work against the tide for so many years, and it nearly pulled me under. I stopped that self-defeating madness. Expectations erode relationships by chipping away at individual self-discovery. Tyler may not agree, but I feel I failed as a parent in this respect. I can say today that I learned from that failure and spend my time since then celebrating him instead of expecting anything.

When talking to my counselor, a thought occurred to me. I told her, "I know Tyler won't lose a moment of sleep or ever second-guess moving away from me, even for a minute. He'll do whatever he's being driven to, and I want him to do just that."

"Even though he would move away without concern for you, do you doubt that he loves you?"

"Not for a second," I said.

Ah-ha! Detachment with love came to life. I had to accept yet another cliché. "You mean, If I did virtually anything for myself without regard for him or his consideration, he would never question my love for him?" I asked.

"No, why would he?" She said. "You're on your own paths, and that has nothing to do with the love you have for one another."

I needed to hear this.

Lesson Nine: Find Gratitude

Even though they could have, these experiences haven't killed me; they have given me an abundance of empathy for others. These experiences have shown me patience and kindness. They have shown me the makings of unconditional love. They have shown me that judgment is a disease of its own and they have given me the opportunity to help others. Ultimately, I have seen how little I really know. Many times, I thought: *You have to be kidding me; this is the life I was meant to have? This is what I was meant to contribute?*

And yet, I crawled out of a well of despair to get to this place. I guess there's something to be said for that. I won't win any awards or get any special recognition, but I am finally at peace with myself and this life, and that is its own reward.

Maybe my most important discoveries are these:

- I can't control his outcome any more than I can control the direction of the wind.
- More than anything, I'm fortunate to have finally discovered that I am simply lucky to be Tyler's mom.
- I'm lucky I am the one chosen to be there for him when he chooses to need me.
- I'm lucky to have learned the lessons he has taught me.
- I'm lucky that I get another hug from him on yet another day.

CHAPTER 25

A MOTHER'S LOVE

> *Ye who suffer because ye love, love still more.*
> ~ Victor Hugo
> *Les Misérables*

Over the last decade, I've read everything I could get my hands on from the perspective of the addict in an attempt to understand just a morsel of what my son had to endure, but I kept searching for the perspectives of those whose experiences most closely connected to mine. I had to know. I wanted to relate to others so I would know I wasn't going crazy. I wanted to know the guilt and shame I was feeling wouldn't swallow me whole but would somehow actually heal over time.

Guilt and shame are not solely laid on the back of addicts. Oh, no—these emotions get to be experienced by all involved. The guilt is often innate to your existence as a parent. I felt guilty if I was having fun, if I was eating, or if I was warm in my bed. I felt guilty if I had a glass of wine. *How dare I drink the poison that is killing my son?* And then the whiplash thought of: *Why shouldn't I be allowed to enjoy a glass of wine? I don't have a problem with alcohol.* I felt guilty for helping and for not helping him. I had days when I was riddled with guilt for the way I raised my son, for choices I made or didn't make.

And then, for no particular reason, I stopped having so much guilt. I came to understand that guilt is a feeling developed out of the past. If we knew then what we know today, we would likely have done things so much differently. I was simply doing the best I could with the knowledge I had at that time and not with the knowledge I now have. This concept took a long time to sink in.

It's possible that discussing my feelings directly with my son helped alleviate some of those destructive emotions, but the impetus was likely learning that someone else had stolen my son's trust and ability to feel safe, and that someone wasn't me. It didn't give me a pass for my participation and past mistakes, nor did finding causation provide some sort of correlation, but it helped make sense of the bigger picture.

My son's alcohol abuse disorder began before he experienced trauma. But I believe the trauma became the catalyst for his life's undoing. All the life-altering devastation began happening after 2012. 2012 was the year he was raped by a university football coach.

Our relationship crossed the threshold of healthy early into my son's addiction and went straight to the realm of a debilitating codependency. A perfect example was when I found myself sleeping at his apartment literally to watch whether he'd continue to breathe through the night. I question how I got through many days, and some, I nearly didn't. It felt chaotic every day. I attempted to will the illusion of some better outcome into existence with the preoccupation of my son's survival, but it's like taking my power source and giving it to a false idea. I was the one losing the power and becoming weaker each day. I got good at attempting to control the things I thought I could instead of the one I knew I never would be able to. I used whatever imaginable outlet I could find to help distract me from my reality and to help fill a bottomless void:

- I wrote.
- I walked.
- I isolated.
- I screamed.
- I cried and cried and cried—oceans.
- I ignored.
- I avoided.
- I got too involved.
- I acted like nothing was wrong.
- I acted like everything was wrong.
- I compartmentalized.
- I tried to work with compassion fatigue.
- I overslept or just stayed in bed.
- I stared at the ceiling instead of sleeping.
- I ate too much.
- I starved myself.
- I tried to enact change.
- I painted ugly paintings.
- I watched mindless television.
- I went shopping and purchased useless things.
- I read and read and read some more.

- I drove around for hours.
- I participated in group therapy.
- I participated in volunteering.
- I avoided any kind of participation.
- I cleaned until I couldn't clean anything else.
- I prayed and prayed and prayed.
- I drank.
- I decayed.
- I almost died.
- I tried to control a disease.

My addiction to false control was parallel to my phone addiction. It was the one constant I had in my relationship with my son. As long as he had a phone, I could talk to him or find him, or control him with all of my wisdom and information. One of the best pages I read in *Guts,* by Kristen Johnston—an absolutely fabulous read—was the list of all the possible addictions we can have. The cell phone was not on that list. Maybe that was due to the book being written in 2012, before cell insanity took hold.

I became obsessed with keeping my phone on, carrying it to every unimaginable place—the bathroom, the shower, the restaurant, to bed—just in case, of course. I actually answered my son's call in the middle of performing a pap smear. I had the excuse ready too: *I need to be available for my son because he's likely in crisis.* Bullshit. It became my pacifier.

I wish we could go back to the phones on the wall, answering machines, and call waiting. It was simple. When you weren't home, you didn't have to talk to anyone. We didn't know what we didn't know, and that meant ignorance was bliss. Now we know everything there is to know at any second of every day, and it creates chronic anxiety.

Just think about how our relationships have changed as a result of the immediate availability this technology has provided. I feel like Pavlov's dog, classically conditioned to the notifications. *Ding!* My dopamine is off to the races, and a mixture of curiosity, fear, dread, and hope wash over me. It's an actual sensation in my body, and it is not normal. We've done this to ourselves, of course, and it's a whole other soapbox issue. It has played a powerful role in the transmission of fear and anxiety in relation to my son's addiction.

Today, I am able to walk away or turn off my phone at night. Sometimes, I have to make a conscious decision to do so, however. It's a game of mental gymnastics every time. Now I am better about letting myself off the hook—pardon the pun. If I miss his call, then that's just the way it is. It's the way it was when I was growing up, when phone anxiety didn't exist.

The love for my son and my addiction to control forced me to spend an entire decade trying to provide him with every imaginable resource I could. This was an effort in futility because in my mind, I convinced myself that if anything ever happened to him, at least I knew I did everything I could. I was only trying to make myself feel better. Was I essentially hurting him to soothe myself in the event he didn't make it?

Our relationship remains strong and connected to this day. He's my beautiful child. He knows we love him unconditionally, and he knows we support his sobriety. He knows we will help him if he asks in healthy ways that encourage continued abstinence from alcohol and drugs. We have philosophical discussions from time to time and talk about typical-life things now. He's got a girlfriend to attend to and a life of his own. This is as it should be, and a more normal relationship with his parents as he has become a man. However, I still felt like there was a race happening and either the trauma or the disease could win in the end.

I've always turned to the phrase; *the only way out is through*. If he fights through the trauma, he may be resurrected—but if the alcoholism wins, the trauma will eat him alive. I can't win the fight for him. I swore, I thought I could. My desperation thought all my decisions could be willed out of emotions such as guilt and fear instead of logic.

People pay me to fix them, so why wouldn't he listen to me as well? Every time I provided my infinite wisdom, I was essentially saying: *I don't think you can do it.* I thought I was coming from a place of love and care, but in reality, I needed to stop telling him what to do, how to do it, and when it should be done. I'm good at telling people what to do—it comes so naturally. I'm a natural-born fixer extraordinaire. And how lucky was he to get my unsolicited advice?

Not lucky at all, it turns out.

I finally recognized that I had continually given Tyler a pass on his substance use out of empathy and what I thought was love for him and because of my guilt. After I learned about the trauma he experienced, I felt completely powerless to interject my desires for his sobriety because the tide was simply too strong. The rape was the rip current, and I had no life jacket. All along, I was simply absorbing his consequences so that he didn't have to feel any more pain. In reality, I was perpetuating it.

It was probably an unfair burden for my son to be an only child. He was the focus of all our attention. Maybe it felt like a microscope was focused on his life at times, although that was never the intention.

I just want an adult relationship with my son today: the one where he calls to tell me about a new job or a new puppy he and his girlfriend got together. The one in which I'm not perpetually worried or in which I'm excited to see his name come up on my phone instead of dreading something has gone terribly wrong. The kind of relationship in which I didn't know he was hurt so badly in his past and that he'll carry that memory forward through all of his days. I learned to stop letting hope bleed too far into the future.

CHAPTER 26

PEACE

If you don't leave your past in the past, it will destroy your future. Live for what today has to offer, not what yesterday has taken away.

~ Unknown

It only took me fifty-two years to figure out how to live in the right now.

I've always been able to believe tomorrow would be better. Maybe this is because the sum of my disposition has always been gratitude. It likely comes from my spirituality; I was born with this as the core of my being, and somehow my son was too.

Even though there are no guarantees that my son will make it, as I said before, I thank God for another day on this Earth with him. I wake up grateful for sight, smell, health, and a soft bed. I'm aware of the warmth of a shower, my puppy's adorableness, and the smell of coffee in the morning.

There's never a moment when I'm not aware of the things I have. Sometimes that can feel heavy, but humility and gratitude have given me the ability to impart strength to endure this trial my husband and I have been handed. Is there any way you can see yourself finding gratitude in the midst of your loved one's addiction?

There will be incredibly dark days, but you always have to make the conscious effort to come back to awareness and healing. I am aware how difficult that can be when you're faced with the tragedy of loving a person who is addicted, but if you build a solid foundation of strength, wherever you can find it, you will be able to build your life again.

I finally and begrudgingly realized that attending to him without adjusting my own oxygen mask first was either going to suffocate us both or leave only one of us with the ability to breathe. I was trying to give him what little oxygen I had left for so long, I failed to realize I was out of air.

Our entire journey with Tyler's addiction led me to seek strength in unfamiliar places, which ironically led to more peace in my life, and I so desperately want that for you too.

I discovered scientists diligently working on research in the field of addiction and learned there's hope for a brighter future for people with substance use disorder. I learned about new therapy modalities that have great potential for recovery. I learned new ways to communicate effectively, so that transformation could actually happen. I also began examining the multiple religious pillars to gain deeper understanding and discover what purpose this all had. These are aspects that can hopefully give all of us light in the darkness. But in one particular Hindu scripture, known as Gita, I learned a valuable life lesson that I may not have happened upon otherwise. I hope it can help you who are struggling in the darkness as well.

I learned that according to the scripture, there are higher and lower values. Higher values propel and elevate us toward happiness, fulfillment, and meaning. Lower values demote us toward anxiety, depression, and suffering. Higher values and qualities are fearlessness, purity of mind, gratitude, service and charity, acceptance, performing sacrifice, deep study, austerity, straightforwardness, nonviolence, truthfulness, absence of anger, renunciation, perspective, restraint from fault finding, compassion toward all living beings, satisfaction, gentleness/kindness, integrity, and determination. The six lower values are greed, lust, anger, ego, illusion, and envy. Today, I make every effort to attain and live by the higher values. By doing so, I feel I release that energy toward my son. No one chooses to live in the depths of anxiety, depression, and suffering, but you can make the choice to live with the higher values imprinted on your heart every day.

Today, Tyler is in remission, but the reality is we're in a continuum that I have no control over. That is what I have come to understand and, ultimately, accept. I've had to accept that remission is not a guarantee, and there is no cure. Guarantees and cures are things that happen in the future, and I refuse to go there. Today, this day, he is happy and healthy and alive, and I am grateful for today.

Each story is written differently. That is real life. My son has had unwavering aspirations all along this winding path. They are his aspirations, not mine. That's better than okay, and now I am finally able see how wonderful his own personal hopes and dreams are.

The monster in my son's life might have derailed those aspirations for a time, but Tyler's bullish disposition fought and continues to fight. It has kept him alive despite his illness.

Do I still worry? Of course I do. What mother doesn't to some degree? Sometimes I've wondered how I have remained standing. How did I continue to take care of others in my practice while my world was crumbling down around me? We all have to acquire an overriding numbness at times to protect our fragile system. It's what humans do. They persevere and remain resilient. I'm not in any way giving up the fight, but I have to prepare myself for the possibility that this doesn't end like a fairy tale. I imagine it is the same for anyone with a loved one who has been diagnosed with an incurable illness.

I have not been able to put my pain on display before I started expelling it here, but I've come to understand and truly relish the benefits of this release. I feel as if someone excised a 200 pound tumor. I can move around more freely without the straitjacket I had bound myself in. I hope you will find your release as well.

Maybe there are those who are fortunate enough to have to overcome nothing. My son and our family are not in that lucky pool of people, yet we are stronger, wiser, and even more grateful because of it. I couldn't be a prouder parent for raising a son who has managed to survive against more odds than most would ever have to face. We can cut ourselves off from actualization if we choose to do so, but I'm glad I didn't because I needed to grow. I hope that I have. I have been able to let go of the judgments that were not serving him or me. I have accepted that I am Tyler's mother, and I was never meant to be his savior, his keeper, his God, his decision maker, nor his complicit friend.

This experience has changed my identity and I finally understand that I am not my son's addiction.

I was and remain:
- A wife
- A daughter
- A physician assistant
- A sister
- A friend
- An animal lover
- An amateur music connoisseur
- A writer
- A singer
- A not-half-bad cook
- A dancer
- A dreamer
- A photographer

and so many more things, *including* a mother. These parts of myself are valuable and meaningful and fulfilling.

I wasn't, and I'm still not, willing to give up the most important thing I have left. I have taken up residence in the hope state, even though the cost of living there is the highest of anywhere in the world. I don't plan on moving anytime soon. Hope has to be the last thing we ever lose.

Love yourself.

Cherish your loved one and the time you have with them.

xoxo

EPILOGUE

During what I felt at the time was the godforsaken last decade of my life, I was always able to visualize my free-spirited self across an imaginary bridge.

I could look across and see she felt good and alive over there. I was always smiling and hopeful, yet I couldn't get to her. I desired her life more than anything else. It was the life I had before this evil plague entered my world—the life full of innocence, naivety, and blind bliss. Instead I remained on the side with the impending monsoon ready to wipe me out over and over again. I stayed and prayed for understanding and enlightenment for my son, but it actually came to me instead.

Each prayer, each experience, each person I met in the storm was a step across that bridge. I now look back and see my former self. She's defeated, shriveled, and devoid of self-love. She is full of doubt, guilt, and fear, and she's aging at warp speed.

She's so alone.

If there is such a thing as hell, I believe I've already been there. It's where I was on the other side of that bridge. I existed there for entirely too long. I'm not there anymore.

ACKNOWLEDGMENTS

Life has shown me so many things, and it dared me to recognize the good that exists in the universe. I have met sympathetic police officers and nurses who showed my son dignity and showed our family compassion. They've renewed my faith in their professions. I am eternally thankful for them.

I also want to express gratitude:

To the organizations that were there when we needed them most, such as Trillium and NAMI, the National Alliance on Mental Illness: their work with mental health and substance use disorder communities continues to be lifesaving to so many.

To the male inmates of the Sheriff's Heroin Addiction Recovery Program for their courage and willingness to work with me. I appreciate how much they taught me about real humanity.

To the entire team at Capucia Publishing for your support and for keeping me moving forward with this terrifying and humbling effort. And to my editor, Heather Taylor, for your exceptional skills and patience with me. You helped me to sculpt a block of clay and turn it into a story I hope will help someone else. You were the vital tool I needed to give myself the confidence to do this.

To our office staff for their constant willingness to adjust my schedule time and time again and for their understanding when I wasn't always the most pleasant person to be around, thank you. A special thank-you as well to Brenda, the office guru and miracle worker, for your endless words of encouragement.

To the patients who accepted those schedule changes, and especially to the ones who shared their family's own personal heartache of addiction: we bonded in unique ways, and I am so grateful we connected with one another.

To our dear friends who didn't run for the hills when they saw us coming and stuck with us through thick and thin: a very special appreciation goes to Julie, Kris, Doug, Ginny, Trent, Nusara, Steve, Fernando, Frances, Mike, Mary, Prudencio and Leslie—you mean the world to us.

To my mom and stepdad, Wade, for your willingness to help in some of the most difficult situations and to deal with my heartache over the years: thank you for always being at the other end of the phone and caring for Tyler in some of the most difficult situations.

To Debbie and Carol, for being willing simply to listen when I needed you most. You both are more a part of my heart than you'll ever know.

There were those who suggested I write a book after hearing my story, but my dearest appreciation goes out to Elissa for not only encouraging that I write this, but for remaining a dear friend throughout the entire process, forever cheering me on.

To my husband for being my constant. I never had to worry if you would be there, even though I didn't want to put you through it. Your support and your love for Tyler and me made it possible to do this.

To my courageous son for allowing me to tell your story so that we may help others. Thank you for baring your soul to me so that we were able to grow in the ways we most needed to.

ACKNOWLEDGMENTS

Some of the most beautiful people in the world are the fellow addicts, parents, and other loved ones we've met on our journey. Their hearts were always on their sleeves, and it created the most beautiful and vulnerable connections possible. Nothing binds you to others quite like the frailties of the human experience.

REFERENCES

Duke University. 1999. "Exercise May Be Just as Effective as Medication for Treating Major Depression." *ScienceDaily* 27, October. sciencedaily.com/releases/1999/10/991027071931.htm

Grisel, Judith. 2019. *Never Enough: The Neuroscience and Experience of Addiction*. London, UK: Scribe.

Oppel Jr., Richard A. and Jugal K. Patel. January 31, 2019. "One Lawyer, 194 Felony Cases, and No Time." *New York Times*.

Perry, Bruce, and Oprah Winfrey. 2021. *What Happened to You? Conversations on Trauma, Resilience, and Healing*. New York: Flatiron Books.

CONTACT THE AUTHOR

✉ admin@lisagennosa.com

🌐 www.lisagennosa.com.

in Lisa Gennosa

ABOUT THE AUTHOR

LISA M. GENNOSA lives in Tarboro, a small, rural town in eastern North Carolina where she is a practicing physician assistant. She is a dedicated wife and mother who grew up the third child of a liquor and narcotics agent turned attorney. Her breadth of exposure to healthcare, the legal field, and parenting an addict provided the foundation to reveal the things we least like to talk about, but most need to. Lisa has conducted countless speaking engagements for police, parole and correctional officers, paramedics, nurses, and other hospital staff in an effort to create positive change. Her son remains the biggest gift in her life.

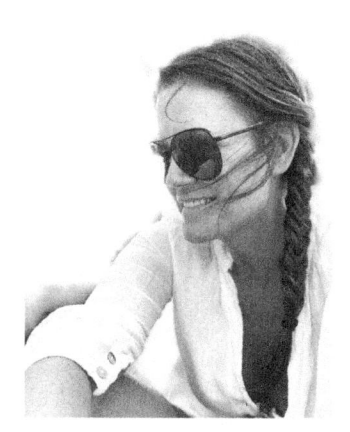

Made in the USA
Las Vegas, NV
04 April 2024